# Sprouted Vegan:

## Your Guide to Plant-Based Health

By Jody Ortiz

## DISCLAIMER

THE AUTHOR IS NOT A DOCTOR AND MAKES NO CLAIMS AS A MEDICAL
PROFESSIONAL. ALL ADVICE AND INFORMATION CONTAINED IN THIS
BOOK IS THE AUTHOR'S OPINION BASED ON RESEARCH AND HER OWN
PERSONAL EXPERIENCE. PLEASE CHECK WITH YOUR PHYSICIAN
BEFORE CHANGING YOUR DIET OR MAKING CHANGES TO YOUR DAILY
SUPPLEMENTS AND MEDICATION. ALL EFFORTS HAVE BEEN MADE TO
ENSURE ACCURACY IN THE INFORMATION PROVIDED IN THIS BOOK.
THE AUTHOR AND PUBLISHER DISCLAIM LIABILITY FOR ANY
OUTCOMES FROM APPLYING METHODS DISCUSSED IN THIS BOOK.

A Haute Books Ink exclusive.

ISBN-9798792776159

Cover Artwork by:
Chelsi Nicole

Interior Design by:
Jody Ortiz

Edited by:
Kathie Giorgio

Pictures in chapter 7 by:
Brandi Price Photography

Adobe stock photos licensed and labeled with artist name

"The earth affords a lavish supply of richness of innocent foods, and offers you banquets that involve no bloodshed or slaughter; only beasts satisfy their hunger with flesh, and not even all of those, because horses, cattle, and sheep live on grass." Pythagoras

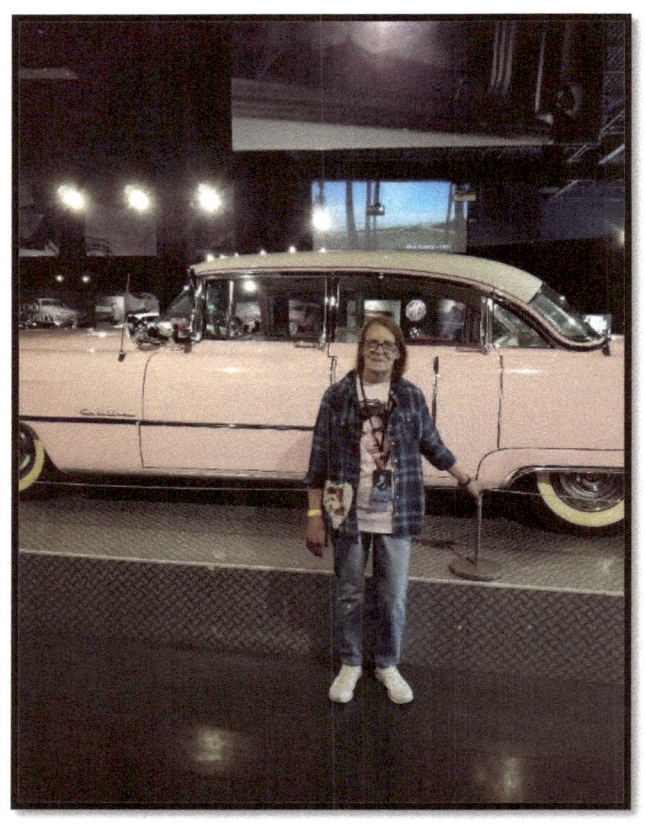

*Mom at Graceland just a few months before she forgot my name.*

*We finally made it to Graceland, Mom!*

# DEDICATION

To my mom, the biggest Elvis fan I know, I miss our conversations and all the fun adventures we shared. I wish I had this knowledge before dementia claimed your mind. Maybe I could have helped you since you taught me about rising above any situation and never giving up. I'll always love you.

To my husband, thank you for your patience and support. You're my rock in more ways than one and you changed my world for the better.

To my daughter, Chelsi, my miracle child to whom miracles occur naturally. Thank you for choosing me to be your mom and for providing me with lessons in unconditional love and strength and support.

To Kathie Giorgio of All Writers, your tireless energy and patience took this book to the next level. Thank you!

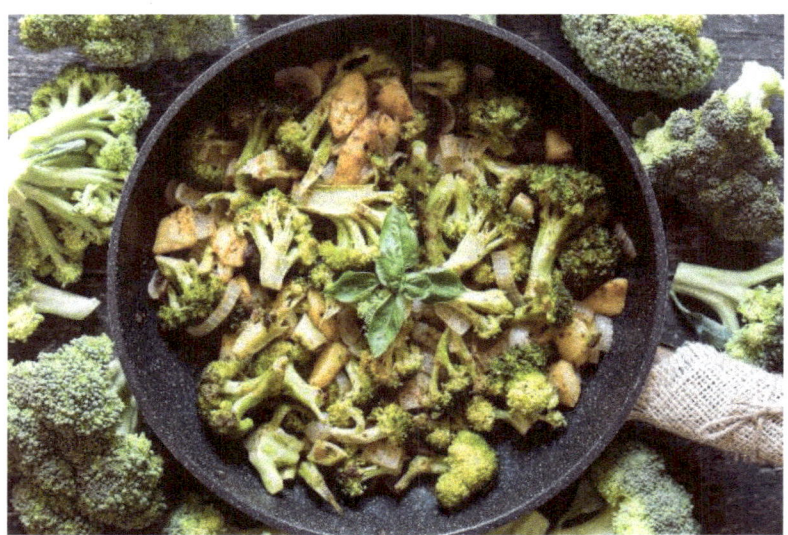

*Picture by RomanWhale Studio*

# CONTENTS

I'M HAPPY YOU'RE HERE     9

THERE IS HOPE     13

STANDARD AMERICAN DIET (SAD)     21

WHAT'S A PLANT-BASED VEGAN DIET?     41

YOUR HEART     49

CANCER     61

WHAT YOUR DOCTOR WON'T TELL YOU     65

HEALING FOODS     68

CHRONIC ILLNESSES     109

DRINK WATER, NOT MILK     113

NO OIL IS HEALTHY     139

THE ENVIRONMENT     153

SUMMARY & CONCLUSIONS     161

GOING PLANT-BASED     163

FOOD SOURCES     166

MAKING THE SWITCH     169

CHEF SECRETS     179

RESTAURANTS     201

ONE WEEK PLAN     207

BONUS HOLIDAY RECIPES      243

RECIPES      260

INDEX      333

SOURCES      336

# I'M HAPPY YOU'RE HERE

*"My body will not be a tomb for other creatures."*
*Leonardo da Vinci*

Was your childhood dream to become plant-based or vegan?

When your mom forced you to eat bacon to "get enough protein," did you put your little five-year-old hands on your hips, raise your chin, and proudly announce, "When I grow up, I'm gonna be a vegan!"?

Probably not. Otherwise, you would have already made the switch.

Changing how you eat, such as deciding to switch to a plant-based or vegan lifestyle, is a decision that often comes after you've received a worrisome diagnosis. It's like a wake-up call nobody wants to hear, but it lights something inside that says, "It's time to get serious about getting healthy," and that means ending your toxic relationship with meat.

If you're like me, someone who grew up eating animals that were raised in our pasture, you know what's on your plate and you're somewhat familiar with how it's turned into food. Even so, throughout your lifetime, it seemed natural to eat it.

You rationalized it.

*Eating animals is the norm.*

*Everyone eats meat.*

Not anymore. Times are changing.

Couple the current state of our overall health as a species with today's level of awareness of what we put into our bodies, and, at some point, and without seeking, you'll have an epiphany. Even if it didn't occur when you were five, it's going to happen, eventually. You might not act on it right away. It could hit you like a bolt of lightning or develop into a slow simmering sensation over months or years. You'll likely continue to eat meat long past your revelation.

But, one day you'll be reminded that the bacon on your plate and the ham between slices of bread in your lunch sack were once living, breathing, feeling, and caring life sources. Then suddenly, the epiphany will break through the rationalizing self-talk and the thought of turning your body into "a tomb for other creatures," as Leonardo de Vinci so eloquently described, will make you want to hurl. It happens, and it's okay that it took a while to get there. We all have our own journey. When I quit meat, it wasn't for the love of animals. It was for my health. I still craved meat, and you will too.

The good news is that reading this book is the first step in changing your destiny.

I can help you.

I've been in your shoes.

My life had to change for health reasons.

I never planned to become a vegan. I didn't think it was healthy or possible, yet here I am. I haven't eaten meat since 2013, and I'm still alive and healthier than ever. You can do it too.

You can improve memory, alleviate pain in your joints, reverse some diagnoses, fit into a smaller size, and help save animals and the planet by making a kinder, healthier choice.

People are changing their lives every day, and so can you.

I'm here to hold your hand and answer all your questions. If I don't answer your questions, reach out to me. I'd love to hear from you.

I'm going to be your support system and your biggest cheerleader. I believe in you.

Let's get started!

It's time to introduce you to the new _____ (fill in the blank with your name.)

Your new, healthier, more energetic life starts now.

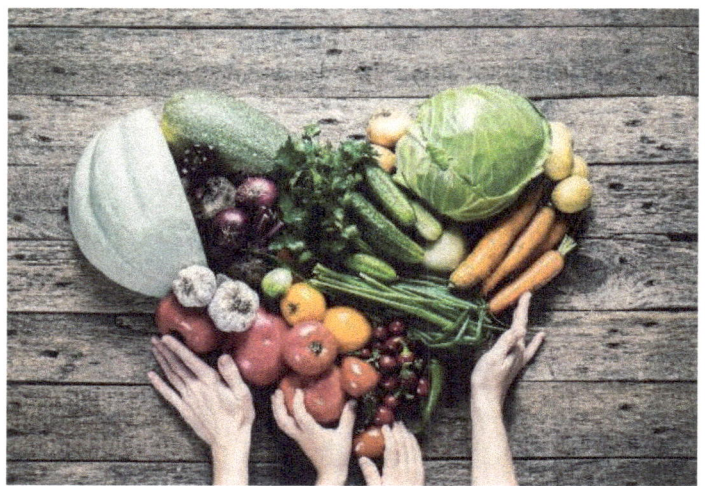

*Picture by olga pink*

# THERE IS HOPE

*"You may encounter many defeats, but you must not be defeated."* Dr. Maya Angelou

As you're aware, issues such as obesity, heart disease, diabetes, depression, and prescription drug addiction plague humanity. It sounds daunting and as if we're doomed to fail as a species. Don't lose hope! There could be a solution to these issues, and it comes from natural sources.

Our planet is rich in every nutrient that our bodies need to survive. But modern-day society has gotten away from turning to nature for nourishment and, instead, we're slowly killing ourselves by eating processed foods and drinking sugar-saturated chemical-laden drinks instead of water. This only adds to the problem and makes people turn to drugs to get healthy instead of learning how to optimize a vegan plant-based diet for their benefit.

Just a couple of generations ago, with our grandparents and great-grandparents in the post-depression era, the appreciation for plants in our diet diminished.

Our great-grandmothers prepared meals from ingredients grown on their home farms or bought at local mills and ranches. My maternal great-grandfather owned one of those mills, as well as a farm. My paternal grandfather fed his family only what he grew in his garden or caught in the nearby lake.

For those older generations located in the Midwest and in other farming areas, their food was local, fresh, and didn't include chemicals. It also wasn't heavily processed. It was healthy food grown by weathered hands that plowed fields, planted gardens, harvested crops, shucked corn, snapped green beans, dug up potatoes, canned summer vegetables, churned butter, milked cows, plucked chickens, and gathered eggs. Every meal was not a feast of animal-based products.

They ate eggs when the hens laid. They ate beef when the cow was mature enough to butcher. They ate pork after the hog feasted on what was left in the garden after the summer harvest and was fattened. They ate butter when they had a cow to milk and after spending hours churning. They worked hard to eat, and their diets consisted of whatever was available to them. Even those in large cities had access to imported grains, vegetables, and legumes that were canned, and meats that were cured, but not heavily processed like today's foods.

For those of us who didn't come from a lineage with servants in our households, our great-grandmothers spent most of their days preparing and cooking foods and cleaning their homes. Their jobs were laborious and time-consuming, which meant they were more active and naturally burned more calories to stay healthy.

When processed and pre-canned foods became available, their children - our grandmothers - were liberated from the kitchen. They changed how they fed their families and instead of snapping green beans and digging up potatoes, they opened metal cans and poured the pre-salted foods into a pan, added store-bought butter and refined salt, heated the food, and served it to their families, alongside a main meat dish. Meals became heavily salted, processed, and animal based.

All my maternal grandmother's recipes in her old church cookbooks list a can of this and a box of that and, consequently, she was the first generation in our family to find it necessary to join Weight Watchers. For as long as I can remember, she struggled with her weight, along with type 2 diabetes, though she was never large by today's standards. At a size 12, she would be considered average today.

Mom's weight was always an issue as well. She also purchased a can and box of everything to go along with the meat from an animal that fattened in our pasture or Dad killed in the wild. Every night, we ate one green and one yellow canned vegetable, and a canned biscuit, along with the hamburger or tuna mix in a box, or a piece of meat. During the summer, we ate food from the garden. I preferred the canned food I ate at Grandma's to fresh garden vegetables. As a child, I thought Mom didn't know how to cook. Her food didn't have the same texture as the canned food, and it was bland without all the added salt. I can remember several nights when I went to bed hungry because I refused to eat my dinner.

I wish our grandparents knew that while they were freeing themselves from the kitchen, they were, in some cases, creating health issues for themselves, but mostly for their descendants because of the bad eating habits they passed down to the next generation. Perhaps if they could see into the future, this book wouldn't be necessary. Sadly, that's not the reality we face.

## Plants are the answer

Research has proven that diseases such as heart disease, cancer, and type 2 diabetes can be treated and possibly even avoided through the consumption of low-fat plant-based vegan foods. When dietary options are possible, fewer prescriptions and invasive medical interventions are necessary.[1] By educating not only the public but also medical professionals and dieticians on the life-saving power of plants, we could save money on healthcare costs. We could also experience longer, more productive and active lives with less pain, fewer instances of depression, and, most importantly, less medication, like the reality our great-grandparents knew.

Yes, our grandparents ate meat.

Let's quantify this statement again. They ate smaller portions of meat and less frequently than what is considered today's norm. Meat was a necessary ingredient in some situations in the past. But, as you'll learn throughout the pages of this book, today meat is unnecessary to maintain a healthy diet.

Also, we have more food options. We have grocery stores, farmer's markets, food delivery, Amazon, local farms, and some of us carry on family traditions and grow our own food. We no longer need to wait until something is in season. We can even buy frozen cherries in the winter! Our options are plentiful and I'm going to provide you with a healthy meal plan that is filling, nutritious, and tasty without meat. It can be done. I promise!

I had that moment of "Oh crap! I have to change how I eat!" and began my journey in 2007, but finally switched to full-time meat-free in May 2013. I transitioned into a plant-based vegan diet for my own health reasons. In the process, I became certified in plant-based nutrition through Cornell University's online nutrition program, and I successfully completed both the Forks over Knives plant-based cooking class and the professional plant-based chef class through Rouxbe, an online cooking school.

Along my journey, I erased the multi-generational bad eating habits and healed my body of symptoms from multiple health issues, including rheumatoid arthritis, heart disease, Sjogren's, hypoglycemia, asthma, and lupus. I was too late to prevent a diagnosis of Barrett's esophagus, a pre-cancerous condition that will require monitoring for the rest of my life. Because of changes I've made in how I eat, progression of the condition is unlikely.

Recently, a restaurant served a wrap to me that contained meat. It was supposed to be a falafel wrap. I didn't realize it was meat until I ate a few bites and had an immediate reaction, which included diarrhea and full body itchy hives that lasted for three weeks. My doctor recognized the signs of alpha-gal syndrome and blood tests confirmed the diagnosis. It's a condition caused by a tick bite. Eating animal products, particularly from animals with hair, could literally kill me.

Is alpha-gal evolution's way of turning humans into vegans?

It's an interesting concept and my issues with throwing up when trying to eat meat from 2007 to when I quit for good in 2013 now make sense. I'm allergic!

My daughter was born with food allergies and also grew up eating processed food. She is currently battling a rare "incurable" condition called reflexive sympathetic dystrophy (RSD), also known as complex regional pain syndrome (CRPS), with secondary erythromelalgia, postural orthostatic tachycardia syndrome (POTS), and Raynaud's. Symptoms from RSD attacked her nervous system, causing the signals that go from her brain to her legs to become scrambled, taking away her ability to walk. She is also currently following a plant-based diet as one of the essential forms of treatment and she's making slow, but steady progress. After five and a half years of being bedridden and unable to care for herself, she is now walking short distances and has taken control of most of her daily care. She's living WALKING evidence that miracles do occur and that plants truly hold a healing power.

If our stories resonate with you, don't take this as medical advice. Every body is different and diseases affect people in different ways. I consider my experience with lupus mild compared to some others with the illness and I caught my esophageal issue in time to do something about it before it turned into cancer. Yet, my daughter's RSD is more progressive and difficult to treat than most similar cases. The doctors deemed her "full body, severe."

Every person has a different experience with a diagnosis, so please speak to your doctor about your specific needs. I'm not a doctor, nor am I a medical professional, and I make no claim of authority on health issues. I'm a vegan health coach. My expertise is preparing and eating plant-based vegan foods.

18

Please seek your doctor's opinion or get a second or third opinion before starting any new way of eating or discontinuing medication that is prescribed by your doctor.

In the meantime, strap in, because some of the information in this book may turn your world upside down. I recall the feelings that overcame me when I realized how every bite of food I chose to eat was making me sick. My definition of a healthy meal contained minimal quantities of nutrition, at best. This realization was difficult to swallow, at first.

As time passed and I no longer experienced arthritis pain or threw up or choked on food because I made better dietary choices, I felt more in control of not only my health, but my overall well-being. After learning how to balance a healthy vegan diet and cook whole foods, I'm now confident in the kitchen, and I no longer have pangs of guilt or doubt about my choice to give up animal-based foods. I'm excited to pass on this knowledge and sense of confidence to you. Now it's your turn. Together, we can break the cycle of bad eating and create a better, healthier future for the next generation.

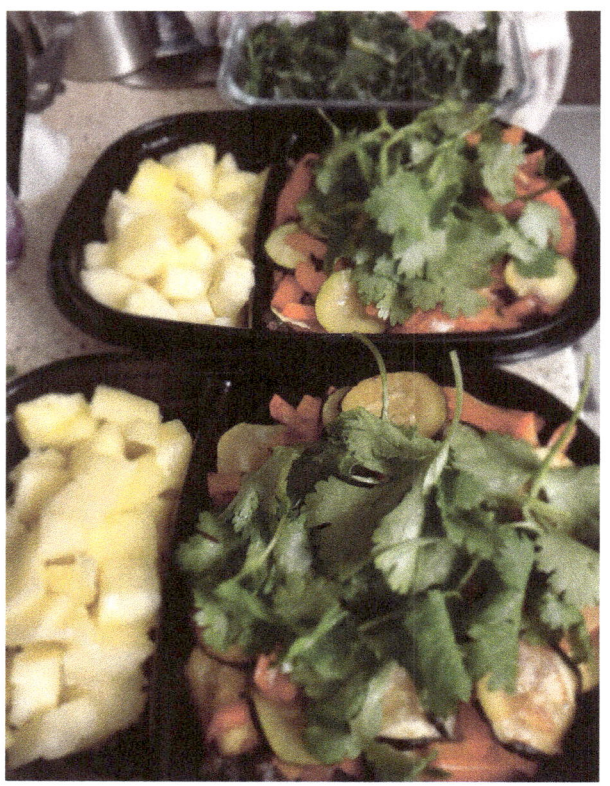

# STANDARD AMERICAN DIET (SAD)

*"If you put junk food in your body, your body will turn to junk." Goldie Hawn*

Within the last few years, the topic of a plant-based whole food lifestyle has been featured in several studies and covered extensively in viral documentaries.[2] Plant-based diets have become a hot button for discussion as the scientific community embraces the connection of nutrition and health.[3] Learning the benefits of using food to treat health conditions is essential to not only those currently facing health concerns, but to future generations as well.[4] Subsequently, scientists, medical professionals, and the awakening general public are searching for available information on plant-based vegan food and its attributed effects on disease and chronic conditions.[5] With the rising level of interest, research is now available, which proves that healing the body and the reversal of certain diseases can occur internally with proper whole food plant-based nutrition.[6]

Living plant-based is nothing new. After the Neolithic period, ancient Egyptians thrived on predominantly plants in what was often a hostile dry landscape. In 2014, the Journal of Archaeological Science published an article entitled "Diet of ancient Egyptians inferred from stable isotope systematics," written by Touzeau et al. that revealed the findings of tests performed on bone, enamel, and hair excavated and collected from mummified heads of Egyptians and Predynastic and Coptic mummies found to inhabit various civilizations throughout the Nile Valley. Animal samples were also tested to explore available food sources within the region and to determine food chain activity. Of the human subjects tested, all but one individual, who is believed to have been a migrant, were consistent in their limited diet composed of locally harvested food of primarily plant-based origins.[7] Archeologists were able to determine the consumption of animal-based protein by testing keratin and collagen levels in the mummies, which was determined to be approximately 19% of their diet.[8] In comparison to today's standards, the average ovo-lacto-vegetarian - someone who eats eggs and dairy products - adds 32% of animal-derived foods to their daily meals.[9] Omnivores, or people who consume both meat and plant-based items, ingest 64% of animal-based foods during their daily regimen. Based on these figures, archeologists determined that ancient Egyptians were predominantly vegetarians. These findings of such an advanced society obliterate the concept that people require animal protein for survival, strength, endurance, and logical reasoning and lend credence to the fact that human beings today can choose to live without it.

Nutritional quality often comes into question in consideration of any type of limited diet. In 2012, in cooperation with a Belgium group known as Ethical Vegetarian Alternative when their name is translated into English, a team of researchers launched an online survey that gathered data from 1,475 participants who listed their current diet type such as vegetarian, vegan, pescatarian, and omnivore, with 104 qualifying as vegan.[10] Participants also listed their sex, current age, height, and weight, giving researchers an indication of their body mass index or BMI.[11] Omnivores represented the largest class of overweight responders at 20.6% with 8.4% obese, while vegans represented the lowest weights, with only 8.4% overweight and just 1.9% obese. Participants ranked 52 items in a food frequency questionnaire on the number of servings they ate per day over a span of one year. Their responses were broken down into the total number of nutrients consumed on an average day. The study found that vegans ranked highest on the Healthy Eating Index while omnivores had the lowest ranking. Vegans also had lower protein and sodium levels and higher amounts of dietary fiber and healthy fats with a low intake of saturated fats. Additionally, vegans consumed higher amounts of fruits and vegetables than any other group of responders. The researchers concluded that the vegan diet was the healthiest in terms of nutritional values.

**Where do you get protein?**

The first question vegans and vegetarians are asked by curious or concerned omnivores is where we get our protein. According to the Daily Recommended Intake calculator provided by the United States Department of Agriculture, the recommended daily allowance of protein for a 50-year-old female of average height and weight is 58 grams.[12] Clarys et al. found that vegans consume on average 82 grams of protein per day, which is 41% higher than what is recommended, given the parameters in the above example. Therefore, protein sources are plentiful in a vegan diet with options such as legumes, nuts, nut milks, soy products, and so on.

The Choose My Plate campaign promoted by the United States Department of Agriculture claims that one ounce of nuts or one cup of legumes is equal to the same amount of protein found in two ounces of shrimp or six slices of lunch meat, making getting the daily recommended amount of protein an achievable goal without animal product consumption.[13]

## Vegan for health

A Gallup poll conducted in 2012 reported that only 2% of Americans polled identified as vegan.[14] A similar poll conducted six years later in 2018 reported 3% of respondents as vegan.[15] Not much has changed. Since most Americans follow an omnivore diet, throughout this book I will provide research to back up my belief that the nation is experiencing a nutritional crisis by eating animal-based products.

In an effort to provide data on the connection of diet and health, Dr. Joan Sabate, a board certified physician who specializes in internal medicine and serves as the Executive Director of the Center for Nutrition, Lifestyle, and Disease Prevention at Loma Linda University, along with Lap Tai Le, research coordinator and adjunct professor at California State University, San Bernardino, conducted a study of peer-reviewed articles published on Seventh Day Adventists that covered their dietary habits and reported health.[16] Their research pooled data from 96,000 Adventists with 48% omnivores, 28% lacto-ovo-vegetarians, 10% pescatarians, 6% semi-vegetarians, and 8% vegans. From their pooled data, they discovered that vegans have a 78% risk reduction for diabetes, a 14% risk reduction for all cancers, and vegan males experience a 42% risk reduction in cardiovascular disease mortality and a 55% risk reduction in ischemic heart disease. Sabete and Le concluded that vegan diets help to deter chronic conditions and diseases such as cancer, cardiovascular mortality, hypertension, obesity, and type 2 diabetes, with added benefits in some cases for male vegetarians and vegans. Their research provides a roadmap for the most beneficial dietary choices and overall health.

Since 1938, more Americans have died from heart disease and cancer than any other cause, not including deaths from Covid-19.[17] A search online provides information about numerous health issues such as heart disease and cancer that can be reversed and prevented through diet. Research studies determined that vegans have a 55% lower chance of heart disease and a lower risk of Type 2 diabetes, if a healthy plant-based diet is followed. [18],[19] The lack of nutritional education provided to doctors is adding to not only the decline in healthcare,[20] but also to the cost of diseases nationwide.[21] Proper nutrition not only effects the body, but also mental health.[22] For all the stated reasons, the benefits of a plant-based vegan diet should be discussed as a viable solution before medication or surgery. A vegan plant-based diet provides the nutrition a human body needs to not only survive, but also to heal.

## History of the American diet and its dependency on processed foods and animal products

Since the start of mankind, humans have been resilient in nourishing their bodies through foraging, hunting, gathering, trading, and growing their own food. They survived on instinct and information passed down for generations on what was safe to eat and what to avoid. As Charles Darwin discovered when studying the wildlife on the Galapagos Islands, survival of the earliest humans was instinctual and necessary for the end goal of breeding and passing on strong traits to offspring.[23] Throughout history, life was difficult during droughts and times of starvation, but simple in choosing what to eat. Humans ate when hungry and when food was available. They did not follow dietary guidelines on how much and what types of food are necessary to sustain themselves. They felt hunger and ate something. Simple. People followed primarily whole food plant-based diets with the addition of meat when available and without concern for inadequate nutrition or pressure from governmental agencies and advertisers to eat certain foods. They followed their own instincts and ate what was available to them and how much their bodies told them they needed to eat.[24]

## Eat plants not supplements

Flash forward a few million years to today's complicated dietary recommendations. Vitamin and supplement companies spend big bucks on advertising to convince us all that we aren't getting adequate supplies of nutrition from food. They convince us that we need to supplement our diets with pills, shakes, powders, and snacks.

In 2011, the multi-vitamin market alone raked in $11 billion.[25] The supplemental market reported selling $28 billion in 2010.[26] According to the National Health and Nutrition Examination Survey, between the years of 2003 and 2006, 40% to 50% of Americans over the age of 50 used a multi-vitamin supplement as part of their daily regimen. With such booming business, it seems that research would support the need for these costly dietary additions.

However, in 1994, the Alpha-Tocopheral Beta-Carotene Cancer Prevention study gave over 29,000 Finnish middle-aged male smokers a form of vitamin E supplement, along with beta carotene. The results astounded researchers with an increased rate of lung cancer of 18% and 8% total mortality from ischemic heart disease and cancer. Instead of helping, the added supplements were found to have worsened the conditions of those affected.[27]

Farin Kamangar with the Department of Public Health Analysis, School of Community Health and Policy, Morgan State University, and Ashkan Emadi from the Department of Medicine, Division of Hematology at John Hopkins School of Medicine surmised that while multi-vitamins increase the chances of diagnoses of certain cancers and heart disease, their placebo effects satisfied those who took them, so their popularity would undoubtedly continue unnecessarily. Kamangar and Emadi stated, "The results of large-scale randomized trials in the past two decades have shown that for the majority of the population, MVM [multivitamin/mineral] supplements are not only ineffective, but they may be deleterious to health." [28]

Vitamin E is often touted as a wonder drug. It's given credit for preventing cancer, heart attacks, strokes, and other health issues. Savvy online marketers claim it can prevent blood clotting and plaque buildup. Researchers are setting the record straight. The Physicians' Health Study II enrolled 14,641 male doctors over the age of 50 in the United States with low rates of smoking and with reported exercising at least once per week in a study and gave them vitamin E, vitamin C, and a multivitamin. They checked in after a period of 8 years. The update showed 1,943 total cases of cancer in the participants and that the use of vitamin E had no effects on reducing the risks of cancer, including prostate cancer, or on major heart episodes, and hemorrhagic strokes. There were a total of 1,245 major cardiac events after 8 years. An update on the study at around 11.2 years showed minimal difference in the placebo and control group in the usage of a multivitamin, with 1,732 total cardiac events at that time. [29]

The Women's Health Study was led by Buring and Lee of Harvard Medical School and studied 39,876 women aged 45 and older with no serious health concerns. At the end of the 10-year study, it was determined that neither vitamin E nor B-carotene had any significant effects on the reduction of either cancer or cardiovascular events.[30]

## The United States government promoted unhealthy eating habits

Sadly, dietary recommendations are ever-changing as new diet fads flood the market, informing people to avoid gluten, supplement with omega 3, and add even more protein to an already protein-overloaded system that includes animal-based proteins, which are proven carcinogenics.[31] Though guilty of creating a market with what seems to be scare tactics, vitamin and supplement companies do not carry sole responsibility for the ongoing confusion and misinformation. Historical graphics show that the United States government promoted animal-based foods as well as processed foods as an example of a healthy diet.[32] In their "Eat a good breakfast to start a good day" campaign, the Bureau of Human Nutrition and Home Economics listed seven food groups for optimal health. The first three food groups included standard fruits and vegetables. Food group number four started the downward trend with the recommendation of cheese and ice cream plus three to four cups of milk for children per day. The recommendations worsened with group number five listing meat, poultry, fish and eggs, with dried peas and beans as alternatives to the meat products. Food group six included bread, flour, or cereal, adding that they can be whole grain, enriched, or "restored." Group seven tipped the unhealthy scale by promoting butter and fortified margarine as healthy foods.

This misinformation was given without educational supplements on portion sizes or nutritional values for products such as white rice and bleached flour, only adding to the inevitable demise of our nation's health.[33] The following attached image in figure 1 provides an easy-to-follow chart for the United States Department of Agriculture's seven basic food groups.

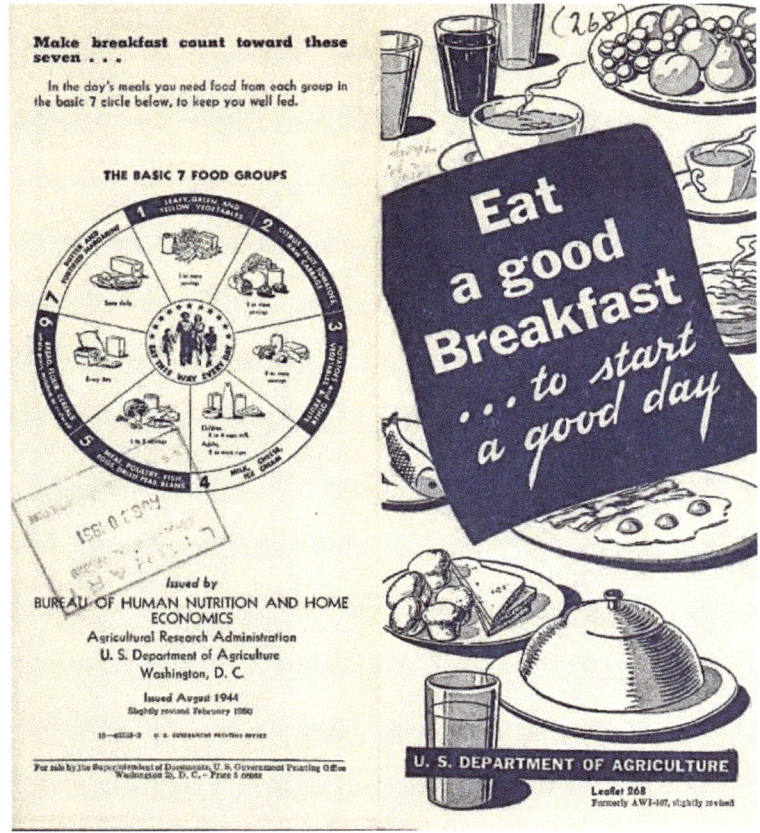

Make Breakfast Count (Ward, 1937, p. 1)

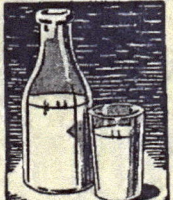

Milk is part of a good breakfast. It's hard to get enough calcium—important mineral for good bones and teeth—without a regular supply of milk in meals. Same is true about the B vitamin, riboflavin—milk is one of the best sources, and a good source of protein as well.

Normal, healthy adults need a pint or more of milk in some form each day. Children should have a quart, if possible.

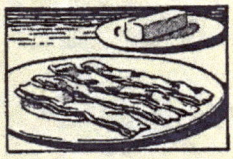

The fat in the spread for your bread or in fat meat helps breakfast to stick to your ribs. That's because fat digests slowly and stays by you longer than most foods.

*Make Breakfast Count (Ward, 1937, p. 3)*

By the early 20th century, scientists were beginning to understand how the bodies of some individuals could not properly break down carbohydrates, which led to symptoms of diabetes. Since white rice is pure carbohydrates and its consumption can contribute to the development of type 2 diabetes, this information should have been shared with the public when promoting white rice as a healthy food choice.[34] With billions of dollars in revenue at stake for supplement and vitamin companies, the misinformation and false advertising will continue, and unsuspecting consumers will pay with not only their finances, but also their health.

## What is the standard American diet (SAD)?

The standard American diet, also known as SAD (a fitting acronym), consists primarily of processed food and animal products.[35] With busy lifestyles and fast-food options on every corner, we're all hooked on junk and we're not getting the recommended daily allowances of plant-based foods.[36] Processed foods taste better, last longer, and are considered a more cost-effective option than whole foods. In lieu of eating an apple or choosing a salad and giving our bodies the nutrients needed, we tend to choose processed foods and reach for advertised supplements in the form of a pill or powder for nutrition. This trend is creating issues within the healthcare system and shortening lifespans. Instead of listening to lobbyists for meat and dairy industries and promoting unhealthy choices such as white rice and foods loaded with saturated fats, the United States government could become a catalyst for change, if only they would embrace the concept of a healthier America.

## Your SAD body

According to the Center for Disease Control and Prevention report in 2016, the leading cause of death at the time was heart disease, with cancer at a close second.[37] These tragic conditions have been attributed to many factors, such as genetics and plain old bad luck, yet scientific research has revealed that what we choose to eat is often the overlooked and undervalued culprit.

The Standard American Diet has spread worldwide with the globalization of American-born fast-food franchises. What were once historically healthy cultures that thrived on plant foods such as whole grain rice and vegetables, and only used minimal servings of meat, primarily as a flavoring agent or a side dish, have adapted our way of eating. Standard diets now include highly processed foods, greater quantities of animal products, fat, sugar, and oil, with rice and vegetables pushed to the side.

The Office of Disease Prevention and Health Promotions reports that three-fourths of Americans do not consume enough fruits and vegetables, but instead stuff themselves with extra protein, sodium, sugar, and fat.[38] Fruits and vegetables, along with other plant products, provide our bodies with essential nutrients as well as dietary fiber to keep waste from building up in our systems, which can cause devastating effects.

According to The National Academies of Sciences Engineering Medicine, men age 50 or younger should consume 38 grams of dietary fiber, per day. Men age 51 and older - 30 grams, women age 50 or younger – 25 grams, age 51 and older – 21 grams.[39]

The following chart is provided online from the Office of Disease Prevention and Health Promotion and lists common sources of dietary fiber from whole foods. [40] Notice there are no animal products on the list because they do not contain dietary fiber.

Dietary Fiber: Food Sources Ranked by Amounts of Dietary Fiber and Energy per Standard Food Portions and per 100 Grams of Food

| Food | Dietary Fiber in Standard Portion | Dietary Fiber per 100 grams |
|------|-----------------------------------|-----------------------------|
| High fiber bran ready-to-eat cereal | 9.1-14.3 | 29.3-47.5 |
| Navy beans, cooked | 9.6 | 10.5 |

| | | |
|---|---|---|
| Small white beans, cooked | 9.3 | 10.4 |
| Yellow beans, cooked | 9.2 | 10.4 |
| Shredded wheat ready-to-eat cereal | 5.0-9.0 | 9.6-15.0 |
| Cranberry (roman) beans, cooked | 8.9 | 10.0 |
| Adzuki beans, cooked | 8.4 | 7.3 |
| French beans, cooked | 8.3 | 9.4 |
| Split peas, cooked | 8.1 | 8.3 |
| Chickpeas, canned | 8.1 | 6.4 |
| Lentils, cooked | 7.8 | 7.9 |
| Pinto beans, cooked | 7.7 | 9.0 |
| Black turtle beans, cooked | 7.7 | 8.3 |
| Mung beans, cooked | 7.7 | 7.6 |
| Black beans, cooked | 7.5 | 8.7 |

| | | |
|---|---|---|
| Artichoke, cooked | 7.2 | 8.6 |
| Lima beans, cooked | 6.6 | 7.0 |
| Great northern beans, canned | 6.4 | 4.9 |
| White beans, canned | 6.3 | 4.8 |
| Kidney beans, cooked | 5.7 | 6.4 |
| Pigeon peas, cooked | 5.6 | 6.7 |
| Cowpeas, cooked | 5.6 | 6.5 |
| Wheat bran flakes, ready-to-eat cereal | 4.9-5.5 | 16.9-18.3 |
| Pear, raw | 5.5 | 3.1 |
| Pumpkin seeds, whole, roasted | 5.2 | 18.4 |
| Baked beans, canned, plain | 5.2 | 4.1 |
| Soybeans, cooked | 5.2 | 6.0 |
| Plain rye wafer crackers | 5.0 | 22.9 |
| Avocado | 5.0 | 6.7 |

| | | |
|---|---|---|
| Fava beans, cooked | 4.6 | 5.4 |
| Pink beans, cooked | 4.5 | 5.3 |
| Apple, with skin | 4.4 | 2.4 |
| Green peas, cooked (fresh, frozen, canned) | 3.5-4.4 | 4.1-5.5 |
| Refried beans, canned | 4.4 | 3.7 |
| Chia seeds, dried | 4.1 | 34.4 |
| Bulgur, cooked | 4.1 | 4.5 |
| Mixed vegetables, cooked from frozen | 4.0 | 4.4 |
| Raspberries | 4.0 | 6.5 |
| Blackberries | 3.8 | 5.3 |
| Collards, cooked | 3.8 | 4.0 |
| Soybeans, green, cooked | 3.8 | 4.2 |
| Prunes, stewed | 3.8 | 3.1 |
| Sweet potato, baked in skin | 3.8 | 3.3 |
| Figs, dried | 3.7 | 9.8 |

| | | |
|---|---|---|
| Pumpkin, canned | 3.6 | 2.9 |
| Potato, baked, with skin | 3.6 | 2.1 |
| Popcorn, air-popped | 3.5 | 14.5 |
| Almonds | 3.5 | 12.5 |
| Pears, dried | 3.4 | 7.5 |
| Whole wheat spaghetti, cooked | 3.2 | 4.5 |
| Parsnips, cooked | 3.1 | 4.0 |
| Sunflower seed kernels, dry roasted | 3.1 | 11.1 |
| Orange | 3.1 | 2.2 |
| Banana | 3.1 | 2.6 |
| Guava | 3.0 | 5.4 |
| Oat bran muffin | 3.0 | 4.6 |
| Winter squash, cooked | 2.9 | 2.8 |
| Dates | 2.9 | 8.0 |
| Pistachios, dry roasted | 2.8 | 9.9 |
| Pecans, roasted | 2.7 | 9.5 |

| | | |
|---|---|---|
| Hazelnuts or filberts | 2.7 | 9.7 |
| Peanuts, roasted | 2.7 | 9.4 |
| Whole wheat parantha bread | 2.7 | 9.6 |
| Quinoa, cooked | 2.6 | 2.8 |

Now let's compare the nutrients in 500 calories of plant-based foods vs. animal products. The plant-based food calculations are based on equal parts of tomatoes, spinach, lima beans, peas, and potatoes. The animal-based food calculations are based on equal parts of beef, pork, chicken, and whole milk.

| Nutrient | Plant-Based | Animal-Based |
|---|---|---|
| Beta-carotene | 29,919 | 17 |
| Calcium | 545 | 252 |
| Cholesterol | 0 | 137 |
| Dietary Fiber | 31 | 0 |
| Fat | 4 | 36 |
| Folate | 1168 | 19 |
| Iron | 20 | 2 |
| Magnesium | 548 | 51 |
| Protein | 33 | 34 |
| Vitamin C | 293 | 4 |
| Vitamin E | 11 | 0.5 |

As you can see, better nutrition comes from plants.

## Complex carbs

Complex carbohydrates are also important to our well-being. Colonic health suffers on extremely low carbohydrate diets such as the Atkins or Keto diets, in which meal plans consist of high fat and low carb foods. The reported ratios on diets such as these are as follows: carbohydrates – 9%, protein – 29%, and fat – 62%. The Institute of Medicine's acceptable macronutrient distribution ranges are carbohydrates – 45% to 65%, protein – 20% to 35%, and fat – 10% to 35%.[41] By inverting these numbers and feasting on extreme amounts of fat with minimal carbs, butyrates have been found to be significantly decreased in fecal samples. This can be detrimental to the human body, considering the profound effects that butyrates have on gene expression, the interpretation of genetic code in DNA. This topic is discussed in more detail in the cancer section of this book.

If you're unfamiliar with the term, a butyrate is a short chain fatty acid (SCFA) that is present in a healthy gut and is produced by probiotics inside the colon. Naturally occurring probiotics are created when fiber in plant-based materials, primarily undigested carbohydrates or complex starches and fibers ferment within the gut and develop into butyrate, also called butyric acid. Butyrates are critical in keeping the body in balance and preventing duplicate harmful cells from forming as cells die, guiding cells in the process of cellular regeneration and preventing the formation of colorectal cancer as well as ulcerative colitis.[42]

Butyrates also help to control inflammation within the colon along with the inflammatory response in autoimmune disorders. Butyrates likewise are potentially helpful in cases of insulin resistance and ischemic stroke, among others. By limiting plant-based foods and complex or resistant carbohydrates, you are essentially putting yourself at risk of experiencing health issues throughout your body, with symptoms such as headache, constipation, muscle cramps, and general weakness, and increasing your risk of mortality.

Complex carbohydrates do more than aid in creating short chain fatty acids. They are also used in some areas of healing within the mainstream medical field. Resistant starch and hydration are vital in treating children effected by V. cholerae to stop diarrhea and help in recovery. These resistant starches or complex carbohydrates are found in foods such as oats, rice, potatoes, and legumes, to name a few. [43]

In one documented case, a 36-year-old man adapted the Atkins diet and was successful at losing weight by eating 1/3 of his normal amount of white rice and eating meat daily along with 5 servings of minced or processed meat per week. Within a year and a half of adopting a high fat, low carb lifestyle, he noticed blood in his stool. A colonoscopy led to a diagnosis of ulcerative colitis. He had no family history of irritable bowel syndrome and had no medical history of surgeries, other than an appendectomy more than a decade prior to his diagnosis. Two years into the Atkins diet he was diagnosed and switched to a semi-vegetarian diet, slowing the appearance of blood, but it did not stop it completely. During an 11-day educational hospitalization, he followed a plant-based diet. The blood was no longer present and his abdominal pain was alleviated. Upon discharge, he was instructed to continue a plant-based diet, but he did not maintain it due to a claim of time constraints. Blood once again appeared in his stools within 10 months of hospitalization. [44]

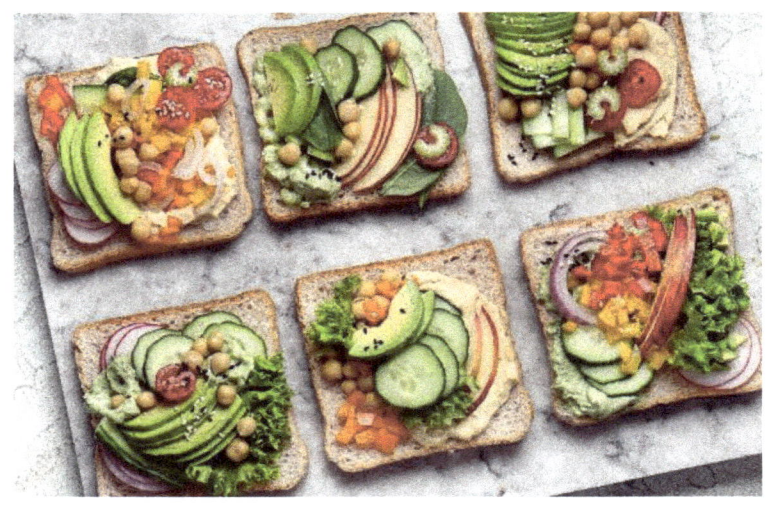

*Picture by Bit24*

# WHAT IS A PLANT-BASED

# VEGAN DIET?

*"If you're not willing to learn, no one can help you. If you're determined to learn, no one can stop you." Author unknown*

A plant-based diet consists mostly of foods made from whole plants with little to no processing, along with a reduction in the consumption of animal-based foods.[45] In general terms, plant-based diets include meat and dairy, but sparingly as side dishes or as a seasoning with legumes and nuts as replacements in most dishes. Those who follow a plant-based diet eat more fruits, vegetables, nuts, and legumes than their omnivorous counterparts. Choosing a plant-based diet is not actually a diet at all, but more like a lifestyle where healthy nutritious choices are favored over what has come to be known as the standard American diet.

## What is the difference between plant-based and plant-based vegan?

The standard vegan diet has just one rule, NO ANIMAL-BASED PRODUCTS. That means no meat, no fish, no eggs, no dairy, and nothing that uses animal parts as a binder or any type of ingredient. You'd be surprised at how many products use animal parts. I used to like gummy bears. But a standard gummy bear is made with gelatin and contains hooves, skin, bones, and cartilage from slaughtered pigs. Think about that the next time you reach for a bowl of Jell-O or your favorite jelly. Even some capsules are made from gelatin, so I always look for the vegan seal when purchasing anything in a package. The good news is that vegan food companies are getting into the market with gummy bear, Jell-O, and fruit preserve options. I actually prefer fruit preserves now over jelly. Try it. You'll like it as well. Since I only take B-12 and the occasional vitamin C or D supplement as needed, I choose the My Kind brand. You can find it on Amazon. It's certified organic, non-GMO, and vegan. The company was co-founded by famous vegan and animal rights activist, Alicia Silverstone.

When someone who is vegan follows a plant-based diet, their focus is not only on healthy choices that come with being plant-based, such as giving up processed foods and white flour, white rice, and sugar, while eliminating oil, but also on consuming only plant-based foods and eliminating all animal-based foods. **This is a plant-based vegan.**

While being vegan is a healthier choice than someone who consumes meat and dairy and it offers nutritional benefits, simply cutting animal products is not enough to ensure optimal health because nutritional gaps must be filled with plant-based foods. To be considered a healthy vegan, a plant-based vegan diet is the optimal choice. Calories consumed come from whole plant-based foods provide more nutrients than processed vegan options.[46]

Dr. T. Collin Campbell is a professor emeritus of nutritional studies at Cornell University. He's best known as the biochemist who blazed the trail in cancer research by studying and publishing his findings on the effects of animal-based versus plant-based protein on cancer patients. According to Dr. Campbell, food is separated into three groups: animal-based foods, processed foods that include fragments of plants, and unrefined whole foods.[47] Dr.

Campbell states that whole unrefined plant-based recipes are self-descriptive and are made from actual plants and not from packaged foods that are processed in a plant, such as cereal or refined pasta. Processed plant fragments also include white rice, white flour, oil, and white sugar because they are refined and not categorized as whole foods, even though they contain trace amounts of plants. Animal-based foods are taken from an animal and can be defined as anything carrying even trace amounts of dairy, beef, pork, poultry, eggs, fish, and so on.[48] These key ingredients in a chosen diet help to differentiate a plant-based diet from a vegan plant-based diet, though they share similarities in focusing on whole plant-based foods as their main sustenance.

Simply choosing a vegan lifestyle does not make one healthy. A healthy vegan is also dependent on the availability of a variety of nutritional food options. In certain geographical locations, access to nutrient-dense foods necessary for optimal nutrition, such as legumes and whole fruits and vegetables, is limited.[49] A plant-based vegan diet is considered nutritionally sufficient only in instances where a variety of plant-based foods are consumed on a daily basis due to the fact that different types of whole foods provide distinct nutrients the body needs. Thankfully, in America and most other developed countries, we have access to the nutritious foods necessary to maintain a well-balanced plant-based vegan diet, unless we're in a food insecure situation. In those cases, supplementation of animal-based foods may be warranted to maintain optimal health. For the purpose of this book, I'm targeting those with access to fresh foods such as fruits, vegetables, and legumes, the staple of my daily nutritional intake.

One of the main drawbacks and concerns in a plant-based vegan diet in cases where access to nutritional supplements are not available is the lack of vitamin B-12 and its necessity to keep a vital neurological system in order, as well as for the formation of red blood cells.[50] Okay. So I stated earlier that supplements are sometimes detrimental to your health and put you at a higher risk of cancer and other issues and they're unnecessary in many cases, but B-12 is the one exception.

Whether a vegan or plant-based vegan lifestyle is followed, in order to maintain optimal health and prevent health-related complications due to nutritional deficiency, a vitamin B-12 supplement must be used and can be taken in pill form, as a shot, or a spray on the tongue.[51] Dr. Thomas Campbell, the son of T. Collin Campbell and plant-based expert, explains the source of vitamin B-12 as a bacterium that does not need oxygen to survive, so it thrives inside an animal's gastrointestinal tract.[52] In the past, humans ingested B-12 naturally with a drastically relaxed concern or care about cleanliness. While it could be said that since humans need B-12 to be healthy and therefore were designed to be omnivores, the evolution of humanity to live in civilized societies concerned with cleanliness would be more of an explanation for the lack of B-12 in plant-based sources than the need to eat animals to obtain a vitamin our ancestors ate naturally.

Today, B-12 intake is rarely a concern for omnivorous humans as they eat animals that naturally eat other animals on the food chain, or the animals eat food that is contaminated with feces, or they just eat their own feces, thereby transferring the bacterium. My husband, daughter, and I went to our local zoo last year and watched a gorilla casually defecate into her hand and then raise her hand to her mouth and….well, you get the idea. Surely our ancestors weren't as unclean, but standards of sanitation have changed tremendously in the past few generations.

According to Dr. Campbell, the average American in a food secure home should not use the scare of a B-12 deficiency as a barrier to jumping into a plant-based vegan diet as it is easily supplemented.[53] A low dose of supplemental B-12 of 2.4 mcg per day is enough. Dr. Campbell suggests the lowest dose possible to maintain the proper level of B-12. A study conducted between the years of 2000 and 2002 concluded that men between the ages of 50 and 76 had a 30% to 40% increased chance of lung cancer after supplementing with vitamins B-6 and B-12, dosing B-12 at .4 mg (400 mcg) per day which is higher than the daily recommended value of 2.4 mcg per day.[54] The study proves that proper B-12 maintenance is possible with minimal supplementation or concern for lack of this essential nutrient. The My Kind B-12 supplement that I use has 500 mcg per spray, offering 8,833% of the daily recommended allowance.[55] When I first started using it, I thought the more the better if it helps with memory and energy and the nervous system and so on. I used two to three sprays. Now I just use a partial spray and I still get more than enough B-12.

In 2014 shortly after going vegetarian, my B-12 was 312 pg-ml, which is low, but not deficient. At this point, I had symptoms of neuropathy in my feet where it felt like the earth was moving and I suffered memory loss. A neurologist diagnosed me within 5 minutes, telling me that her son was vegan and he visited over the holidays and complained of the same symptoms. She prescribed 1 egg per week and chuckled, stating she knew that like her son I would not follow her advice. Instead, I tried several B-12 supplements before settling on the My Kind spray.

```
Tests: (1) VITAMIN B12 (VITB12)
    VITAMIN B12              312 pg/mL              193-982        *1

Tests: (2) FOLIC ACID (FOL)
    FOLIC ACID         [H]  17.6 ng/mL             3.0-17.0       *2

Note: An exclamation mark (!) indicates a result that was not dispersed into the flowsheet.
Document Creation Date: 09/23/2014 3:42 PM
```

My B-12 was tested again in 2017 and had more than doubled to 698 pg/ml and I have no issues with any of the previous symptoms and only use a partial My Kind spray.

```
Tests: (1) VITAMIN B12 (VITB12)
    VITAMIN B12             698 pg/mL              193-982        *1

Note: An exclamation mark (!) indicates a result that was not dispersed into the flowsheet.
Document Creation Date: 01/12/2017 6:21 PM
```

## Why do whole foods provide better nutrition than refined foods?

Whole foods such as rice and wheat are made up of three important components which are bran, germ, and endosperm. When wheat or rice are refined and turned white, both the bran and germ are removed, leaving only starch and endosperm, and also taking away the B1 and B6 vitamins, fiber, magnesium, phosphorus, and selenium. Therefore, refined foods such as white rice and white flour are stripped of their nutritional value during processing and are not considered plant-based foods because they fall into the processed plant fragment category. A vegan plant-based diet focuses on whole foods and grains such as amaranth, barley, brown rice, millet, rolled oats, and whole wheat because they are nutritionally dense foods.

When comparing whole grain to refined wheat, the amount of protein remains the same. However, dietary fiber is reduced from 13% to 3% and sugar is increased from 70% to 83%, increasing the glycemic index and possible contribution to the development of diseases such as type 2 diabetes.[56]

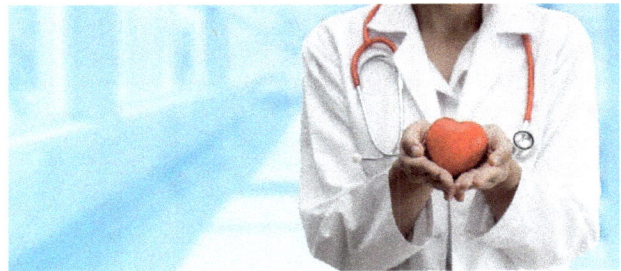

*Picture by Blue Planet Studio*

# Your heart

*"If the truth be known, coronary artery disease is a toothless paper tiger that need never exist, and if it does exist, it need never ever progress."*

*Dr. Caldwell Esselstyn*

In the United States, every 37 seconds, a person dies from a heart disease-related complication. Before Covid-19, this was one out of four deaths.[57] The birth rate in 2018 was one baby every 8 seconds, which counteracted the astonishing rate of death. After the age of 20, 18.2 million Americans or 11.6% of adults over 20 are diagnosed with coronary artery disease (CAD).[58] CAD kills two out of ten Americans under the age of 65. Every 40 seconds, a heart attack occurs in America. These statistics are both frightening and tragic with the knowledge that changing one's lifestyle could prevent such a devastating end.

According to the Center for Disease Control and Prevention, heart disease is caused by the following conditions: diabetes, excessive drinking of alcoholic beverages, high blood cholesterol, high blood pressure, obesity or being overweight, smoking, not following a healthy diet, and living a sedentary lifestyle. The CDC's Division of Nutrition, Physical Activity, and Obesity suggests the following food choices to control heart disease: add healthy fats such as olive oil, top lean meats with avocado, reduce sodium, eat more fiber such as fresh fruits and vegetables, and choose a variety of colors. This information has changed for the better since 1947, but it still promotes oil and animal products, which are not heart healthy as proven in this section.[59]

## Cholesterol

As briefly mentioned previously, there is zero cholesterol in plant-based food. Since there are multiple food products and supplements on the market that promise to lower your cholesterol, you would naturally assume that eating a plant-based diet void of any and all cholesterol is a good choice. For the most part, you would be correct in that assumption. However, your body needs cholesterol to function. Cholesterol reduces inflammation, creates bile acid for digestion, converts sunlight into vitamin D, and provides your body with estrogen and cholesterol, but too much of the bad cholesterol can lead to issues such as fatty liver and plaque. Both of these issues can lead to heart failure or a heart event. Fatty liver occurs when your liver is overloaded with lipids or fat and it cannot process the excess or break it down. When the liver becomes fatty, it can enlarge and take up too much space and compress on your heart. If you're having heart pain, but your heart checks out okay, have the doctor check you for fatty liver.

So, if you're not getting cholesterol from eating plants, how will you get it? Don't panic. Cholesterol is made within your body, in your liver, to be exact. Your body creates all the cholesterol needed, if functioning correctly. Regular health screenings at your doctor's office will reveal if your body is making enough cholesterol on its own. Since my family has a history of heart disease and heart attacks, I watch out for signs of heart issues. Approximately every two years, I request a nutrition and lipid panel screening from my doctor and my cholesterol levels have remained steady since going vegan. Every body is different. So I would strongly suggest that you check with your doctor to ensure that you're getting enough cholesterol after you start any vegan diet. The U.S. National Library of Medicine suggests that people under the age of 45 have their cholesterol checked every five years and older adults every one to two years.

Normal total cholesterol levels are between 140 to 199 mg/dL. Anything over 240 mg/dL is considered in the high range and hypercholesterolemia. High cholesterol can be caused by a number of issues and not just the consumption of cholesterol-filled foods. Even a plant-based vegan can have high cholesterol. It can be caused by a familial history of high cholesterol, atherosclerosis (plaque in your arteries), cholestasis (when your bile doesn't flow correctly from your liver and buildup occurs), diabetes, obesity, and so on.[60]

On February 12, 2014, almost one year after I quit eating meat, but continued to eat dairy, eggs, and occasional fish, my total cholesterol was 221 and in the high range, as you can see in the chart below. My LDL or bad cholesterol was 134 and high, but my HDL or good cholesterol was in the normal range at 61, creating a risk of a heart event of 2.2, over one-half the average.

```
Tests: (2) LIPID PANEL (LIPID)
   TRIGLYCERIDES            132 mg/dL              35-163          *17
   CHOLESTEROL         [H]  221 mg/dL             120-200          *18
   HDL CHOLESTEROL          61 mg/dL               35-80           *19
   LDL CHOLESTEROL     [H]  134 mg/dL              <130            *20
   LDL/HDL RATIO           2.2 Ratio                               *21
         LDL/HDL RATIO                  RISK
            1.47                 One-half average
            3.22                 Average
            5.03                 Twice average
            6.14                 Three times average
```

On March 27, 2019, five years later after becoming vegan for a number of years at the age of 51, my triglycerides were still in the normal range at 121, my total cholesterol dropped to 195 and was in the normal range and my LDL was normal at 109. My HDL, or good cholesterol, was slightly above normal at 62. I eat a lot of foods such as nuts, which increases HDL. My go-to snack is raw almonds. I keep them in a canister on the kitchen counter and grab a few throughout the day. This is a habit I picked up when dealing with hypoglycemia to get enough protein to counter sugar intake. (We'll discuss this further in the book). The most promising number from the test was my risk of a heart event was reduced from 2.2 to 1.8, still slightly over one-half the average, but lower than when I was vegetarian.

```
Tests: (1) LIPID PANEL (LIPID)
    TRIGLYCERIDES          121 mg/dL                    <90           *1
       Normal <150 mg/dL; Borderline high 150-199 mg/dL
       High 200-499 mg/dL; Very high > or = 500 mg/dL
    CHOLESTEROL            195 mg/dl                     <200          *2
       Desirable <200mg/dL; Borderline 200-239mg/dL;High>= 240mg/dL
    HDL CHOLESTEROL   [H]  62 mg/dL                      40-59         *3
       Low <40 mg/dL; Normal 40-59 mg/dL; High > or = 60 mg/dL
    LDL CHOLESTEROL        109 mg/dL                     <130          *4
       Optimal <100 mg/dL; Near optimal 100-129 mg/dL
       Borderline 130-159 mg/dL;High 160-189 mg/dL;
       Very high > or = 190 mg/dL
    LDL/HDL RATIO          1.8 ratio                                   *5
          LDL/HDL RATIO               RISK
             1.47              One-half average
             3.22              Average
             5.03              Twice average
             6.14              Three times average
```

My cholesterol levels changed without the use of any medication to reduce cholesterol and, as you can see, it stayed within a reasonably normal range, even though I did not consume any animal products starting in 2016, three years before this test was conducted.

As I mentioned before, there are two terms for cholesterol, "good cholesterol," which is the HDL or high-density lipoprotein, and "bad cholesterol," LDL or low-density lipoprotein. Contrary to how it may seem, you can't eat good cholesterol. Your body creates good cholesterol from a chemical process that occurs mostly in your liver and it's based on your dietary intake. Bad cholesterol is found in animal products and is created after you consume extra fat that your body doesn't need.

Let's pause for a moment and review the term "lipoprotein," which is significant in this explanation of how cholesterol is developed inside your body, its function, and why one type is good and one type is bad. Lipoproteins are constructed with fat and protein since cholesterol doesn't dilute in liquid, so it must be carried. Lipoproteins carry the cholesterol (lipid or fat) throughout the body in water, fluids, and in the bloodstream. LDL accounts for most of the cholesterol count and a high LDL puts a person at risk for either a heart attack or stroke because it is not eliminated from the body. This causes plaque to then build up on arterial walls which then narrow and block the flow of blood to the heart and organs, a term known as atherosclerosis.

HDL is good cholesterol and you want to increase this number because it absorbs cholesterol in the body and transports it to the liver, where it's eliminated. Your body creates HDL when you consume foods rich in omega-3 fatty acids; the good fat. According to the National Institutes of Health, females over the age of 19 require 1.1 grams of omega-3s per day, while males require 1.6 grams per day.[61] The following chart provides just a few sources of plant-based omega-3s.

| Source | Omega-3 Fatty Acid in grams |
|---|---|
| Black walnuts, 1 ounce | .76 |
| Bread, whole wheat, 1 slice | .04 |

| Brussels sprouts, ½ cup | 44 |
|---|---|
| Chia seed, 1 ounce | 5.06 |
| Edamame, ½ cup | .28 |
| English walnuts, 1 ounce | 2.57 |
| Flaxseed whole, 1 Tbsp | 2.35 |
| Kidney beans, ½ cup | .10 |
| Refried beans, ½ cup | .21 |

As illustrated above, by eating plant-based foods, you provide your body with more than enough omega-3 fatty acids without requiring supplementation.

### Heart failure treatment with a plant-based diet

Heart failure can be prevented and treated with a plant-based diet because it is not only healthy, but also low in fat with no added oil or animal food.[62] This determination was made after researchers compiled peer-reviewed studies of individuals with cardiovascular disease, both in and out of heart failure, who were instructed to follow diets like Dietary Approaches to Stop Hypertension (DASH) and the Mediterranean diet.

DASH was created for omnivores with heart disease. The diet contains animal protein to supplicate omnivores, but with added healthy food choices that include plant foods that are low in fat to attempt to replicate the proven lower blood pressures found in vegetarians. In 2012, 6,814 people without cardiovascular disease reported fewer strokes and better end diastolic volume after switching to the DASH diet. In 2013, after one year on the diet, a group of 144,000 adults saw a 19% reduction in coronary heart disease, a 21% stroke reduction, and 29% fewer instances of heart failure.

The Mediterranean Diet is somewhat plant-based by promoting fruits, vegetables, and whole grains, but it is moderate in fat, which raises the bad cholesterol levels. The Lyon Diet Heart Study proposed that if a Mediterranean Diet were followed posterior to the first heart attack, it could reduce complications. Out of 303 participants over a period of 27 months, eight who stuck with the standard diet of animal products and processed food suffered from non-fatal heart failure, while only two who changed their diet to the Mediterranean plan experienced heart failure. When comparing the DASH and Mediterranean Diet plans, both include animal products, but limit processed foods and red meat. In a study of 3,215 women who experienced heart failure, 16% had a decrease in mortality on the DASH Diet compared to 15% on the Mediterranean Diet. Since both diets limit processed foods and red meat, this could presumably be the contributing factor for the diets' success.[63]

Several years ago, a one-year trial of a low-fat diet with 406 patients who experienced a heart attack and were diagnosed with angina reported significant weight loss, higher HDL, lower LDL and total cholesterol, lower triglycerides, lower blood pressure, stable blood glucose, fewer heart failure events and lower mortality rates. Recently, a similar trial reported 84% fewer incidents of mortality among participants who ate 7% fat in their total daily calorie intake after experiencing their first heart attack. In comparison to DASH and the Mediterranean diets' mortality reduction of 16% and 15% respectively, the low-fat option with a mortality reduction of 84% is significantly higher.[64]

According to Kerley, a low-fat plant-based diet is the only plan that has been proven to not only reduce the risks associated with coronary artery disease, but reverse the disease altogether. After 24 days, 46 CAD patients who switched to a low-fat plant-based diet reported significant increases in exercise capability and lower total cholesterol and angina episodes. After three months, the group reported weight loss and lower LDL and C-reactive protein, a measure for inflammation in the body that heightens the chance of a heart attack, and they maintained the benefits at the one-year review. In all, fruit, soy protein, wholegrains, legumes, fiber, monounsaturated fat, polyunsaturated fat, dietary nitrate, antioxidants such as vitamin C and lycopene, magnesium, and potassium reduced the incidents and severity of cardiac events. Meat, salty snacks, fried foods, eggs, fried fish, sweetened beverages, saturated fatty acids, trans fatty acids, dietary cholesterol, and sodium increased the number of incidents and severity of heart failure.65

## Vegan diets and blood pressure

A systematic review was conducted by researchers of seven clinical trials and 32 observational studies. When conducting such reviews, researchers comb through published peer-reviewed clinical trials and studies and compile the data into a single report of comparable data. This specific review covered a 113-year span, from the years of 1900 to 2013. Researchers compiled information on adults aged 20 and over with the average age of 44.5 for whom a vegetarian diet was used as an intervention for high blood pressure.[66] Every clinical trial and study except one provided food for the participants. Of the trials, two were vegan. The researchers defined a vegetarian diet as excluding meat and including dairy, eggs, and fish, which is basically an ovo-lacto-vegetarian, but for this purpose, we'll look at the emphasis on plant-based foods. After looking through all the findings, the researchers concluded that eating a vegetarian or vegan diet lowers blood pressure with a 14% mortality reduction rate.[67]

Between the years of 2002 and 2007, 96,000 Seventh Day Adventists living in the United States and Canada participated in the Adventist Study 2 (AHS-2). From that study, 500 non-black with 3% Asian individuals were chosen to test their blood pressure and body mass index (BMI). The participants' diets were analyzed, with 40% reported to be omnivorous, 36% ovo-lacto-vegetarian, 14% semi-vegetarian, and 10% vegan with a median age of 62 to 67 and 64% female. The research team found almost zero distinction between the four diet types of those currently taking blood pressure lowering medications. For those without medication, in vegans and ovo-lacto-vegetarians, both their systolic and diastolic ranges were significantly lower than in the omnivores. Researchers concluded that vegans had the lowest range of blood pressure, though the ovo-lacto-vegetarians also showed promising results.[68]

### The American Heart Association: Friend or foe?

The American Heart Association's website is sponsored by several corporations, including Eggland's Best, and they promote foods with cholesterol and fat as healthy choices. Researchers compiled studies on dietary cholesterol from eggs and its effect on humans and found 17 studies that met with their criteria. The studies included data from 422 men and 134 women and their changes in HDL, LDL, and total cholesterol when consuming one egg per day or its equivalent in an egg substitute. The conclusion was that when adding an egg to a daily diet, the cholesterol ratio rose by 0.040 units, which increased the likelihood of a cardiac event by 2.1%.[69] While this number is not significant, most Americans do not consume just one egg, they eat at least two eggs or more, presumably creating an even larger likelihood of a cardiac event. To put it in simple terms, one egg contains 200 mg of cholesterol. The daily recommended allowance is 300mg. Therefore, eating one egg is reasonable, but each additional egg adds to your cholesterol intake for the day and puts you over the daily recommended allowance. So why is the American Heart Association promoting eggs as heart healthy?

A search of the American Heart Association's recipe selection retrieves options such as meatloaf with not only ground beef, but also topped with chicken, bound with an egg, and saturated with cooking spray (oil which is, as you recall, the bad fat). The list of ingredients in one recipe is as follows: dry breadcrumbs, fat-free milk, egg, ground beef, chicken breast, vegetables, spices, and cooking spray.[70] In my opinion, the only healthy items in that list are the vegetables. It's my opinion that an organization such as the American Heart Association should only share heart-healthy options if their goal is to combat heart disease.

### What does your heart hospital's menu tell you?

Just a few miles from my home is a heart hospital. It's an imposing building that sticks out in the otherwise flat landscape of homes and small businesses, and the construction to add on additional wings seems to be ongoing. One of the requirements of the plant-based chef class I took through Rouxbe, a professional online culinary school where I received a certification as a professional plant-based chef, was to look at the menu of a local hospital and offer an opinion on whether or not it's healthy and how it could be changed to make it more appropriate to foster good health and healing. I chose the heart hospital for the assignment.

What I found was that the hospital's menu contains primarily foods that promote heart disease and other chronic conditions as discussed previously. On their menu for November 6, 2019, for breakfast, the choices were scrambled eggs, boiled eggs, biscuits and gravy, ham, hash browns, sausage bites, grits and Cream of Wheat.[71] There were no fruit options and, as discussed, foods such as eggs, gravy, ham, hash browns, and sausage are detrimental to heart patients by adding bad fat to their diets. Foods such as eggs, ham, and sausage are loaded with animal fats, which make them high fat foods that block arteries, and they are not recommended for heart patients. The hospital's biscuits do not designate that they are whole grain; therefore, they're possibly made with processed white flour. In southern states such as Oklahoma, gravy is made with dairy, white flour, and oil. These are all products that add to heart disease. Hash browns are either cooked in oil or butter, adding to arterial blockage. Grits or Cream of Wheat are likely served with milk, butter, and sugar, which are all contributors to heart disease. As a heart hospital, they should be leading the way in educating the public and their patients in what constitutes a heart-healthy diet. For heart-healthy options, they should serve fruit, whole wheat bread, and a tofu scramble with green leafy vegetables, as these have been proven to reverse heart disease when prepared properly (more about this later), along with a cup of decaffeinated tea.

If more Americans learned to increase their fiber intake, eat more plant-based foods, skip the oil-laden products, and eliminate animal products or at least reduce them to a couple of times per week, we would not have heart disease-related deaths every 37 seconds.

# CANCER CAN BE PREVENTED AND TREATED WITH FOOD

*"Don't count the days. Make the days count."*
*Muhammad Ali*

Carl Voit, a famous German scientist in the 19th century, discovered that men only needed 48.5 grams of protein per day. However, since protein is associated automatically with meat consumption and the cattle industry was big business even then, his recommended daily allowance was a shocking 118 grams! Voit's bad advice was passed along to his proteges Max Rubner and W. O. Atwater.[72]

Rubner stated that eating a large amount of protein, i.e. meat, was the mark of a civilized person. Atwater founded the United States Department of Agriculture's first nutrition department where he surpassed his mentor's recommendations by stating that 125 grams of protein was the acceptable daily amount.[73] This ballooned figure would later devastate those who followed the guidelines with a continual growth of cancer, diabetes, and heart disease linked to overconsumption of animal products.

T. Colin Campbell was at the forefront of protein research during the years he earned his PhD from 1958 to 1961, with a goal to generate a high protein product that could end the hunger crisis in impoverished nations. Dr Campbell discovered that when lab rats were fed high amounts of animal protein, they developed cancer, but when fed plant-based protein or low protein levels, their cancer cells stopped growing. Once the lab rats were fed high

61

quantities of animal protein again, the cancer cells continued their growth.[74]

Dr. Campbell founded his research on the process of enzymes and the metabolization of aflatoxin when it enters a cell. When an aflatoxin enters a cell, such as when chemicals or drugs are ingested during the metabolization process, dangerous byproducts are formed that can alter a cell's DNA which causes a cell to be damaged. Dr. Campbell hypothesized that, when consumed, protein distorts the process of the metabolization of aflatoxin, and he was correct. He staggered the diets of lab rats, using 20% protein in some and 5% in others and found that the 5% protein group sharply decreased the enzymatic activity at a rate of 72% less DNA binding, 68% less chromatin binding, and 66% less protein binding so that the process of metabolization of aflatoxin slowed and fewer damaged cells were produced.[75]

There are three stages of cancer which are initiation, promotion, and progression. When a carcinogen is introduced into a human's system, it binds to a cell's DNA, creating a carcinogen-DNA complex. If the carcinogen-DNA complex is left untouched and not repaired by the body's natural defense system, it will divide and create daughter cells and these new cells are damaged and are not healthy cells. This is the initiation stage and it can occur within minutes of the carcinogen entering a body. If allowed to continue, the damaged cells cannot be healed and the process cannot be reversed. Damaged cells can remain dormant until they are turned on and from there, they enter the promotion stage.[76]

Looking at this process from a nutritional perspective, if the person eats cancer-promoting foods, such as animal products or processed food with carcinogens, the dormant gene can be switched on causing the spread of cancer. But if the person eats cancer-fighting foods, such as plant-based foods that have been proven to stop cancer growth, then the promotion stage is halted and the cell returns to dormancy. If the cancerous cells are not stopped during the promotion stage, they begin progressing and spreading which eventually develops into a malignancy with the final stage being death. With this process in mind, if cancer is turned off before it progresses, the patient has a fighting chance. Referring back to his research, Dr. Campbell concluded that a human body only requires 10% of energy from protein, yet the average American consumes 15% to 16% or 70 to 100 grams per day. Since most Americans consume animal products, this puts the majority of Americans at risk for developing cancer.[77]

## Colorectal cancer prevention with a plant-based diet.

Among cancer cases in America, colorectal cancer consistently ranks in the number two position with red and processed meat consumption raising risk, while foods that are high in dietary fiber have proven to reduce risk. Researchers set out to prove that colorectal cancer can be prevented and healed with a plant-based diet by compiling data from a study of Seventh Day Adventists, since they are notorious in their preference to abstain from eating meat. Researchers looked at the responses of 77,659 people using five diet types for comparison which were vegans (those who don't eat animal-based products including meat, dairy, or eggs), lacto-ovo vegetarians (those who don't eat meat, but consume dairy and eggs), pescatarians (lacto-ovo vegetarians who also eat fish), semi-vegetarians (those who eat animal-based products occasionally, like on the weekends), and omnivores (those who eat both animal and plant-based products). There were 490 cases of colorectal cancer at the 7-years and 3-month follow-up. Researchers concluded that vegetarians and vegans had a 20% overall lower risk of developing colon or rectal cancers.[78]

## American Cancer Society

The American Cancer Society is promoted as the leader in cancer research and information, providing lifesaving resources to cancer patients via its website. This organization is believed to be on the cutting edge of information, yet they promote recipes that include meat and dairy products to satisfy their sponsors. The formation of cancer is an often-misunderstood scientific process, but with research available that explains how nutrition turns on and off cancerous cells, one would think that organizations such as the American Cancer Society would be at the forefront of sharing this information. With all the information provided in this chapter about research into the association of diet and how it turns on cancer genes, a group such as the American Cancer Society should share the research and at least allow cancer patients to make a choice in how they wish to treat their diagnosis.[79]

# WHAT YOUR DOCTOR

# WON'T TELL YOU

*"The first wealth is health." Ralph Waldo Emerson*

Education about the difference between whole and refined grains is necessary to help the public make the more nutritionally sound choice.[80] Physicians and dieticians are lacking in education on the nutritional properties available in plants.[81] A survey was given to all medical schools based in the United States for the term of August of 2008 through July of 2009 with 86% of those surveyed responding in some part. While most of the schools required some form of nutritional education, just 25% required a course that was designed to cover only nutrition. Of the respondents, only 27% met the standards in 2004 to require 25 hours of education in nutrition. According to research, the amount of education that doctors receive in nutrition has barely changed over the years, leading to concerns about doctors' knowledge and ability to pass on possible life-saving information to their patients.[82]

Vanita Rahman, an internal medicine physician, faced a wake-up call when a 19-year old morbidly obese female patient requested information on bariatric surgery as a solution to her lifelong issues with weight after having failed at several attempts with diets. As a plant-based vegan, Rahman possessed the knowledge to help the patient with guidance on nutritional and lifestyle choices that would be more sustainable than another diet. Yet she regretted the reality that a short office visit did not provide the necessary amount of time to educate her patient properly on how to make the changes. The doctor sadly resolved herself to the reality that a dangerous surgery is often chosen as a solution instead of nutritional education.

Rahman's frustration led to the development of a 12-week program for patients led by a physician and nutritionist that gave patients the resources to build a strong foundation of a whole-food plant-based lifestyle. Rahman also started a program to provide lunch for area physicians as a way to gain their undivided attention. While the physicians ate, Rahman discussed her program, the health benefits, and reasons why the physicians should pass along the information to their patients. Rahman and her team found that physicians were interested in learning more about the program and voiced regret that they did not previously have the knowledge to guide their patients in healthy nutritious choices. This insight into the need with, not just patients, but also the medical community provided Rahman with the necessary information to seek ways to further educate physicians and the public on her plant-based plan.[83]

While it is understandable that physicians cannot become experts in all medical conditions and topics, dieticians should be able to provide education to their clients about plant-based choices. Yet, registered dieticians in Missouri were asked to rate their knowledge of plant-based options that provide protein. There were 136 respondents and most either did not report any interest in learning more about plant-based options or they admitted to having no knowledge on the topic. Still, they acknowledged that plant-based protein is a viable option. At the end of the study, researchers decided that more training in plant-based diets is needed for registered dieticians within the study group area.[84] In order to make the change to a healthier habit of eating whole plant-based foods with no added animal products, it's necessary for both physicians and dieticians to desire the knowledge and to undergo the training necessary to educate their patients on how to get started and how to eat nutritious nutrient-dense foods.

## The cost of healthcare and chronic illnesses

Treating heart disease is one of the largest non-coronavirus health care expenditures in the world to date, costing Americans $273 billion annually. According to data gathered from 2012 by the Centers for Medicare and Medicaid Services' Chronic Conditions Data Warehouse, on behalf of Medicare beneficiaries aged 65 and older, $96 billion was paid to medical providers, hospitals, and third-party billing services for the treatment of heart-related conditions alone.[85] The average cost per patient was $10,345. For this data, heart disease was defined as "congestive heart failure, acute myocardial infarction, unstable angina/acute ischemic heart disease, and specified heart arrythmias."[86] For the year 2017, the Centers for Medicare and Medicaid Services' Chronic Conditions Data Warehouse reports 5,335,238 Medicare beneficiaries sought treatment for heart failure, 20,916,488 were treated for hypertension, and 10,265,211 had ischemic heart disease. These numbers fluctuated between 2012 and 2017 without a drastic change either way in the number of patients seeking treatment for heart-related issues.[87]

The National Center for Chronic Disease Prevention and Health Promotion states that 90% of America's health care costs go toward treating chronic diseases, with heart disease and cancer leading the charts. In 2018, it was reported that over 859,000 Americans are victims of heart disease and stroke mortality each year, with treatment for heart disease costing $199 billion. Nearly 600,000 Americans die from cancer each year and spend $174 billion on cancer treatment.[88] With the rising costs of healthcare, programs like Rahman's may help to alleviate some of the burden on the healthcare system.[89] This makes nutritional education imperative throughout the medical field so that patients can learn that in some cases they can alleviate their symptoms in part or altogether by choosing healthier food options at every meal.

# Healing foods

Hippocrates famously said, "Let food be thy medicine and medicine be thy food." Hippocrates knew that food was healing, yet if you see a traditional Western family doctor or anyone with an M.D. or D.O. after his or her name, it's likely that you will never be told that foods can help alleviate certain symptoms. Your doctor won't tell you because it's not part of the training in medical school or licensing to become a practicing health care provider. How to prescribe prescription drugs safely and legally is taught in medical school, not how to use garlic to treat a tick bite.

Listen to Hippocrates. Food can either make you sick or it can aide in your healing process. This fact you already know. But did you know that cacao was once used to treat anemia, fever, and bronchitis, or that it has the properties to reduce high blood pressure and high cholesterol?

Here are a few facts about common foods that may surprise you.

## Blueberries

*"Forget who you are and why you're here-all that foolishness. In the woods the bushes are full of blueberries; go and pick some." Marty Rubin*

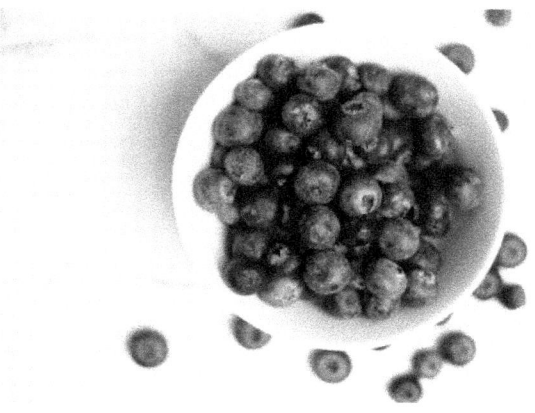

*Picture by Brandi Price*

Blueberries are native to North America in zones five through eight, simply put it's a horizontal strip that extends from the center of North America to the southern states as far as the Gulf of Mexico on the Texas coast and it curves northward on the west coast and fades into Canada. Blueberries were a staple in the Native American diet for thousands of years because of their ability to be stored. In season, they were eaten after picking them fresh off the bush and were also dried and stored for the winter months. Native Americans added blueberries to stews and other dishes and used all parts of the plant including the berries, stems, leaves, and even the roots for medicinal purposes.

Blueberries weren't cultivated, grown on farms, or distributed throughout the country until starting around 1912. In the 1890's, a New Jersey cranberry farmer's daughter, Elizabeth White, saw the benefits of farming blueberries, but nobody else could see her vision or understand how to care for a blueberry plant.

In 1911, a renowned botanist named Frank Coville published a book titled *Experiments in Blueberry Culture* in which he described necessary growing conditions for the plant. Elizabeth White read the book and contacted Coville and offered use of an acre of her farm to cultivate blueberries. Their collaboration prompted the birth of the blueberry industry in America. It took almost a century later for blueberries to be named to the list of superfoods and their popularity exploded.

Today, blueberries are used for treating colic, fever, hemorrhoids, circulation, multiple sclerosis, ulcers, urinary tract infections, and in the prevention of cataracts and glaucoma.

Blueberries are commonly used in baked goods, such as muffins and crumbles and cakes. I add them to a bowl of oatmeal or use them as a salad topping or just grab a handful for a snack. Their versatility makes a tasty addition to every meal. On mornings when I don't have time to prepare breakfast for my daughter, I'll fix a saucer of blueberries, a sliced apple, pear, or peach, and a handful of almonds. It's one of her favorite breakfasts.

Cacao

*"Cacao has great nutritional value, a lot*
*of protein, which strengthens a person,*
*and without sugar it is not fattening."*
Samael Aun Weor

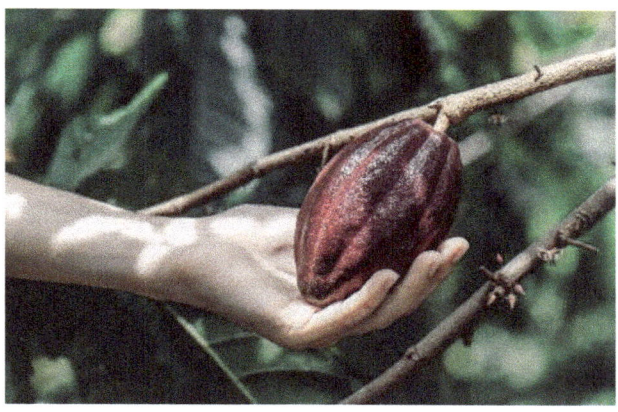

*Picture by Freedom Naruk*

Cacao is native to both the Central and South American forests, but it was first discovered and harvested by the natives of Mexico over 3,000 years ago. They made it into a drink that included chili peppers to add spice. When the Spaniards copied the drink in Europe in the early 1500's, they took away the spice and made it into the sweet drink that we know today as hot chocolate.

It didn't take long for the Europeans to discover the healing properties of cacao and use it in a medicinal setting. By the late 1500's, it was used for ailments such as anemia, bronchitis, fever, and inflammation. Modern scientists have discovered that cacao can be instrumental in treating heart disease because it offers flavonoid antioxidants, such as that in red wine.

71

Cacao has been an instrumental ingredient in my daughter's healing. Every morning, she eats a bowl of pudding for breakfast that I make with both cacao nibs and cacao powder, with cashews as a base. (See the recipe for Cashew Cacao Pudding in the recipe chapter. It's also included in the sample one-week plan.)

Try adding cacao nibs to homemade muffins or cookies. Depending on if you get regular cacao nibs or sweetened nibs, they offer either a bitter or sweet taste along with a welcome crunch.

Cacao is used to lower blood pressure, reduce LDL (bad cholesterol), slow blood clotting to lessen the risk of a stroke, as an antioxidant and anti-inflammatory, and it may help you to survive a heart attack.

## Cinnamon

*"I can't tell you enough about cinnamon. Cinnamon is an awesome spice to use and it goes great with something like apples in the morning or in a mixture of fruit or in your oatmeal or even in your cereal." Emeril Lagasse*

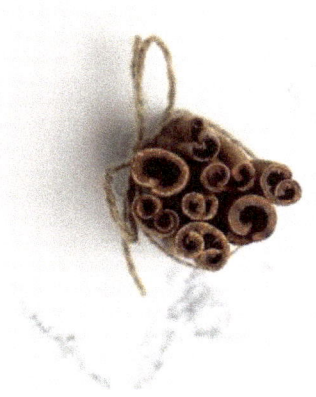

*Picture by Brandi Price*

Cinnamon was prized and traded with a value greater than silver in first century A.D. Rome and was used by only the wealthiest of families. Perhaps the best documentation of its use happened long before Rome in the Bible. Its value was documented in the Old Testament. God told Moses in Exodus 30: 22-29 to use cinnamon to anoint sacred items.

*"The Lord said to Moses, 'Take the finest spices: five hundred shekels of free-flowing myrrh; half that amount, that is, two hundred and fifty shekels, of*

*fragrant cinnamon; two hundred and fifty shekels of fragrant cane; five hundred shekels of cassia-all according to the standard of the sanctuary shekel; together with a hin of olive oil; and blend them into sacred anointing oil, perfumed ointment expertly prepared. With this sacred anointing oil you shall anoint the meeting tent and the ark of the commandments, the table and all its appurtenances, the alter of incense and the alter of holocausts with all its appurtenances, and the laver with its base. When you have consecrated them, they shall be most sacred; whatever touches them shall be sacred.'"*

By the 16<sup>th</sup> century, Europeans recognized the financial potential of cinnamon and took over parts of Asia in hopes of monopolizing the market. As cinnamon became more readily available, the value decreased, and it became a common household spice.

In my kitchen, I use cinnamon for desserts or to create a sweet and savory flavor, such as in my butternut squash soup recipe. I also add a dash of cinnamon to my coffee every morning, along with a spoonful of raw sugar to cut the bitterness of the coffee beans and to control my blood sugar. At lunch, I top salads with crushed nuts dehydrated with a mixture of cinnamon and maple syrup.

In healing, cinnamon is used in Ayurvedic medicine as a digestive aide, but it's mostly used in the West to reduce cholesterol levels and control blood sugar in patients with type 2 diabetes. Cinnamon is one of the few supplements included in my daughter's daily regimen, as RSD is a cousin to diabetes, according to my daughter's specialist, and her symptoms improve when her blood sugar levels are under control.

## Cruciferous veggies

*"Cauliflower is nothing but cabbage with a college education."* Mark Twain

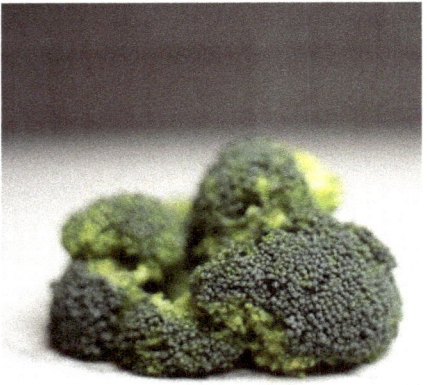

*Picture by Brandi Price*

Cruciferous vegetables are those that are part of the cabbage family. They're called cruciferous because when the plants flower, it has four petals in the shape of a cross, or crucifix.

Examples of cruciferous vegetables are as follows:

Arugula

Bok choy

Broccoli (all versions)

Brussel sprouts

Cabbage (all versions)

Cauliflower

Collard greens

Daikon

Garden cress

Horseradish

Kale

Kohlrabi

Mizuna

Mustard (greens and seeds)

Radish (eat the leaves too)

Rutabaga

Turnips (and the leaves)

Wasabi

Watercress

Cruciferous vegetables have been around for thousands of years and likely originated in Northern Europe in the form of headless cabbages. These plants were then cultivated throughout Europe and Asia before spreading worldwide. If you're interested in reading more about the history, the Triangle of U is a theory written by a Japanese scientist in the early 20th century about the evolution of these plants. It's an interesting concept and has since been validated through dna sequencing.

A common misconception about these vegetables is that they interfere with iodine in the body and can cause thyroid issues. This has been proven untrue. According to Dr. Bakar at Northwestern Medicine, "Cruciferous vegetables are part of a healthy and balanced diet, and I encourage patients with thyroid disorders to continue eating them in moderation. You would have to consume an excessive and unrealistic amount of these vegetables for them to interfere with iodine and thus hormone production in the thyroid."[90]

These foods might not seem appealing if you don't eat a lot of veggies, but they're good for the body. They're high in fiber, contain vitamins C and B9 (folate), and are high in glucosinolates (cancer fighter), potassium, selenium, and phytochemicals. Eating these foods on a regular basis is suggested to reduce your risk of cancers such as breast, bladder, colon, lung, pancreatic, and prostate. They also help to control inflammation, aide in digestion, and help to fight cardiovascular disease. These foods are low in calorie and high in fiber.

In my kitchen, I serve at least one of these foods daily. I make bok choy burritos (see recipes at the end of this book), I sauté kale and add it to Buddha bowls or at the base of salads, I roast broccoli and cauliflower at the beginning of each week in my batch cooking to eat on their own or to put into meals, we eat radishes in salads, turnips in casseroles, Brussel sprouts as a side dish baked with pecans or walnuts, and I stir fry everything and add it to brown rice or quinoa.

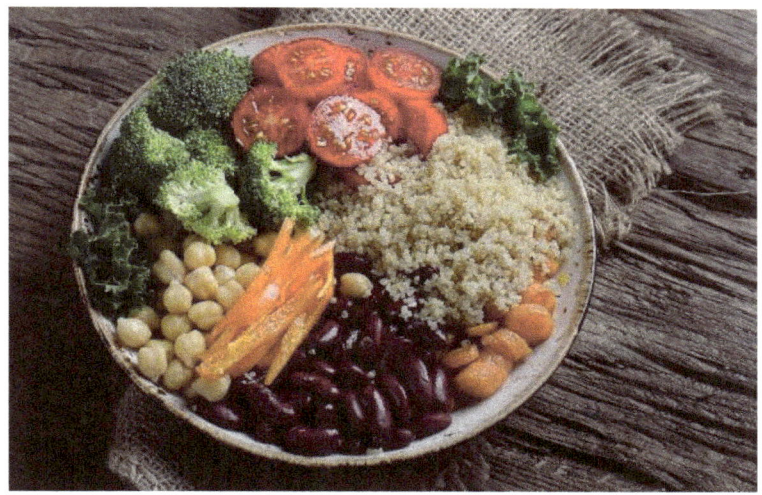

*Picture by Bit24*

# Fennel

*"The fennel is beyond every other vegetable, delicious. It greatly resembles in appearance the largest size celery, perfectly white, and there is no vegetable equals its flavour. It is eaten at dessert, crude, and with, or without dry salt, indeed I preferred it to every other vegetable, or to any fruit."* Thomas Jefferson

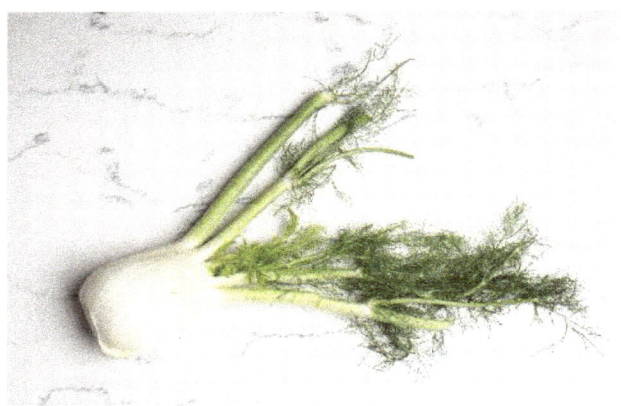

*Picture by Brandi Price*

In ancient Greece fennel was called "marathron" from "maraino," meaning "to grow thin." This was a nod to fennel's natural appetite suppressant properties. Charlemagne touted the healing properties of fennel to Europeans, who later brought it to America when settling the new land. The Puritan settlers used fennel for the same purpose as the ancient Greeks during church services when their stomachs growled from hunger. They referred to the seeds of the plants as "meeting seeds" and discreetly chewed them in church.

Hippocrates prescribed fennel for both mothers and newborns as an herb to stimulate the production of breast milk and to ease the upset stomachs of colicky babies. Ayurvedic practitioners also use fennel for treating stomach issues, and herbalists today continue its traditional use. Fennel is also recognized for soothing sore throats, as a natural cough suppressant, and to relieve stomach cramps.

If you've never tasted fennel, it smells similar to licorice or anise. Fennel seeds can be used to create a soothing tea or even a gargle. The plant can be braised or sautéed to soften the stalk and it can act as an herb in risotto or used in relish, stuffing or potato salad. Chopped finely and sautéed, it adds another flavor component to salads or Buddha bowls. Or, if you're feeling adventurous and want to channel Thomas Jefferson, you can eat fennel for dessert in a rice pudding or fruit tart.

## Garlic

*"Garlic is as good as ten mothers."*

*Les Blank*

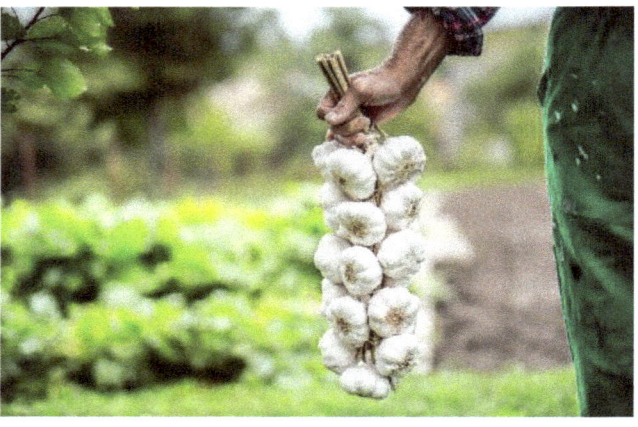

*Picture by Weyo*

Garlic has been used for more than 7,000 years as a source of nutrition and for medicinal purposes and to ensure health and stamina. The slaves who built the great pyramids in Egypt were fed garlic and onions every day so they could keep up with their daily tasks. The Olympic athletes in ancient Greece ate garlic before their competition as a performance enhancer, possibly the first known of its kind. Before antibiotics were used in America, garlic was given to patients to fight off infections.

In my husband's village in Mexico, garlic is ground up and added as flavoring to rice and other traditional dishes, but it's also used to prevent and treat infections. On one trip to Mexico, we just crossed the border and stopped to use the restroom along the toll road and my daughter found a tick on her thigh. We removed the tick, but the area around the bite swelled and itched and irritated her during the remaining twelve-hour drive to my husband's family home. It became so bad that she dragged her leg. After we arrived, my mother-in-law ground up garlic with a mortar and pestle and my husband broke the bite open and he rubbed garlic into the wound. At first, we weren't sure how to react to this seemingly archaic method of dealing with a possible infection. But after two days of the treatment, the swelling subsided and the bite closed up and scabbed over and healed. Now, whenever we get either a tick or spider bite, our first method of treating it is with garlic.

For medicinal purposes, garlic is used for heart disease, to regulate cholesterol, to reduce blood pressure, to strengthen the immune system, and to treat colds, breathing issues, digestion, and cough.

In the kitchen, I add garlic to guacamole, cashew sour cream, dressings, sauces, sautés, soups, and pasta dishes. If anyone in my family feels a cold coming on, we crush the garlic and eat it on a piece of dry toast. There are very few dishes I prepare in which I can't find a use for garlic. It's a staple in my home.

## Ginger

*"I really enjoy making dinner for my
kids and my husband – chopping ginger
and marinating the tofu." Sadie Frost*

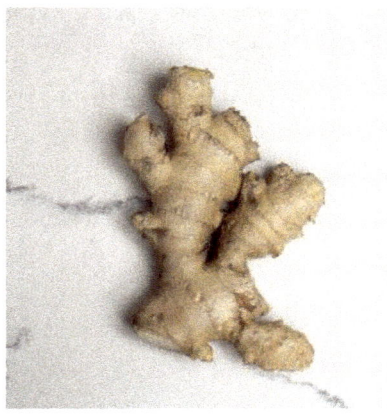

*Picture by Brandi Price*

Ginger's Sanskrit name is vishwabhesaj, which means "universal medicine." It was used in Indian, Asian, Greek, and Arabic cultures as a source of medicine and to treat parasites before being discovered by the Europeans. Its tradition is long with tales from the Middle Ages of its origins in the Garden of Eden.

Ginger is used in the prevention of motion sickness, nausea due to pregnancy, chemo, or food poisoning, for sore throats, cough, cold, flu, headaches, pain and inflammation in arthritis patients, and to treat ulcerative colitis.

I grate fresh ginger into stir fries or mince for a cup of tea. It adds depth to cookie and cake recipes, or you can make your own ginger ale by boiling it in water with raw sugar and adding active dry yeast and lemon.

# Grapes

*"The sun, with all those planets revolving around it and dependent on it, can still ripen a bunch of grapes as if it had nothing else in the universe to do." Galileo Galilei*

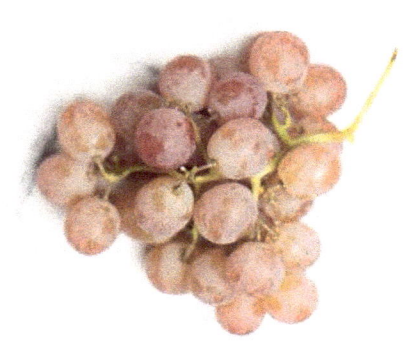

*Picture by Brandi Price*

An archaeological dig of Neolithic ruins in the Democratic Republic of Georgia unearthed pottery jars containing wine residue, dating at around 6,000 to 5,800 BC. Grapes and wine have been used medicinally for thousands of years, even though it's estimated that grape vines were not farmed domestically for 1,000 to 3,000 years after the time period of the ruins. Scholars believe that the grapes used to create the earliest wines were gathered from wild vines, which demonstrates the importance of grapes, even in those early years.[91]

Since grapes cannot be stored for long periods of time in their natural form, one can assume that prehistoric humans used fermenting techniques to turn the grapes into wine out of necessity.

86

In Catholic Mass, wine is used as a symbol of the blood of Christ, a tradition that began with the Last Supper as a memorial of Christ's death and resurrection. In this realm, wine is not only used to heal the mortal body, but to be used as immortal medicine. Jesus said, "The man who eats my flesh and drinks my blood enjoys eternal life, and I will raise him up on the last day." (John 6:54) Since wine became an important part of the Holy Sacraments, its sustainability was ensured throughout the generations.

Herbalists use the entire grape plant for medicinal purposes, creating an ointment from the stem to use for skin issues, and the leaf for bleeding and inflammation. Grapes are used as an antioxidant and to reduce cholesterol, high blood pressure, and coronary heart disease. They help to stimulate circulation and treat coronary venous insufficiency. They're also used to regulate blood sugar, treat eye disorders, and are effective in asthma and allergies.

Whenever I have a sore throat, I crave grapes. They not only add moisture, but they're cold from storing them in the refrigerator and they just make me feel better. Wine has the same affect. As you'll discover in my recipes, I use marsala, sherry, chardonnay, and port wines to deglaze the pan and as a marinade. I choose wines that are in the middle price range with rich flavors, and I use white wine when making white sauces or a creamy roux, and dark wine with mushrooms and in dark-colored sauces.

Raw grapes are one of my favorite snacks, but I also add them to Mediterranean salads and pastas or on top of a fresh summer salad.

## Green Tea

*"If you are cold, tea will warm you; if
you are too heated, it will cool you; if
you are depressed, it will cheer you; if
you are excited, it will calm you."*
*William Ewart Gladstone*

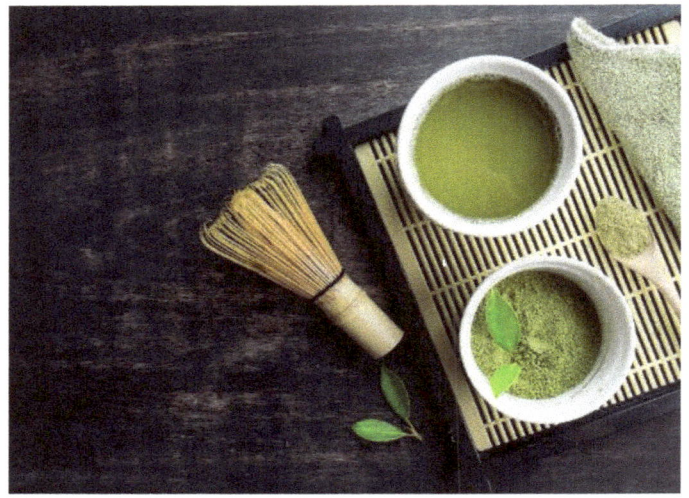

*Picture by Showcake*

The tea craze began in China, though it's unknown as to the exact time period because its origin is surrounded by a mist of myths and legends. Its plant name is camellia (Chinese for "tea flower") sinensis (Latin for "from China"). If left to grow wild, a tea plant will grow into a tree. Tea farmers trim the plants to a height easy to pick, usually resembling a waist-high bush.

The Japanese started drinking tea sometime during the 12th century and it made its way to Europe in the early 17th century. It didn't take long for the English to adopt tea as a national staple, with tea-time rituals that were more about the food than the tea in late afternoons since during this period, only two meals per day were usually eaten. When tea came to America, its taxation sparked the American Revolution.

There are three general varieties of tea which include oolong, black, and green tea. The differences in the types of tea are due to how they are processed. Green tea is unwilted and unoxidized and is scientifically proven to boost health.

In my kitchen, I keep a variety of green teas for everything from sore throats to joint care and stomach aides. If you suffer from heartburn or stomach issues, avoid drinking iced drinks with meals and replace with a warm or room temperature cup of green tea. In recipes, try adding matcha green tea powder to smoothies, vegan yogurts, pancakes, muffins, cookies, and breakfast puddings.

Green tea is used as an antioxidant, anti-inflammatory, to prevent coronary artery disease and cancer, and in reducing cholesterol and regulating blood sugar. For digestion, green tea settles the uncomfortable symptoms of inflammatory bowel disease. Want to lose weight? Green tea is touted as a weight loss secret by boosting your metabolism and burning calories. Experts warn, however, that claims made in the health benefits with the use of green tea cannot be achieved by consuming green tea alone. The effects are most noticeable in conjunction with a change to a healthy diet and regular exercise.

## Leafy Greens

*"Leafy greens such as romaine, lettuce, kale, collards, Swiss chard, and spinach are the most nutrient-dense of all foods."*
*Joel Furman*

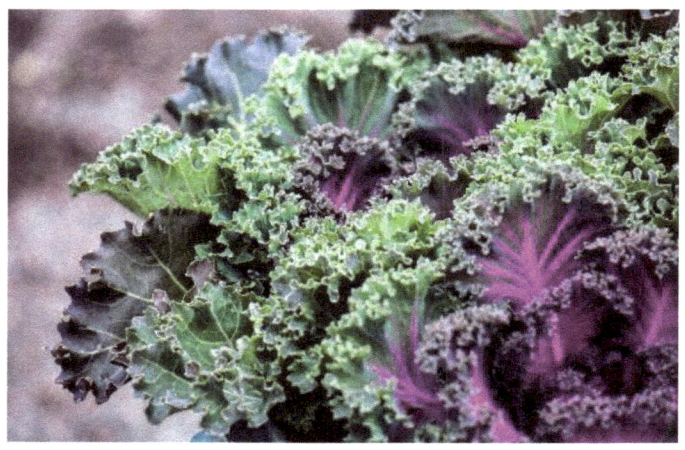

*Picture by Prescott09*

Dark leafy greens are traditionally an African staple, eaten by our prehistoric ancestors before humans migrated around the world. They were imported to America in the 1600s, along with the first African Americans. Leafy greens were woven into traditional southern cooking when enslaved people cooked meals for the white families they served. As the practice of slavery was abolished and the freed people migrated across the United States, they took along with them the dark leafy greens. They're now enjoyed as a staple in all households.[92]

Examples of dark leafy greens are the following:

- Arugula

- Bok choy
- Collard greens
- Dandelion greens
- Kale
- Mustard greens
- Swiss chard

These vegetables are great sources of nutrition, including vitamins A, C, E, and K, calcium, fiber, iron, magnesium, and potassium as well as carotenoids-antioxidants, which play a role in protecting cells from cancer.

My favorite part of dark leafy greens is the fact that they help to cleanse the arteries. Plaque is created from cholesterol calcium, a blood-clotting protein, and waste from cells. The more oily, greasy foods you eat, the more plaque you create, and atherosclerosis or thickened arteries develop because they're caused by a buildup of plaque.

If you're having issues such as high cholesterol, high blood pressure, or erectile dysfunction (ED), eat dark leafy greens daily. Doctors of urology and cardiology refer to ED as a "canary in a coal mine." It's often an early warning sign of blood flow issues. To change your blood flow and start the reversal process, stop eating oil and eat dark leafy greens. (More on this in the chapter on macronutrients.)

In my household, we eat a lot of dark leafy greens. I sauté them and add them to the base of a salad, put them in soups, eat them raw in salads, in wraps, add them to smoothies, and I add them to stir fries. There are so many delicious ways to eat dark leafy greens and none of them involves oil or, as someone suggested to me yesterday, bacon grease. EWWWWW!!

# Peppermint

*"I love peppermint tea, as it's much nicer
than taking anything chemical for
settling your stomach." Deirdre O'Kane*

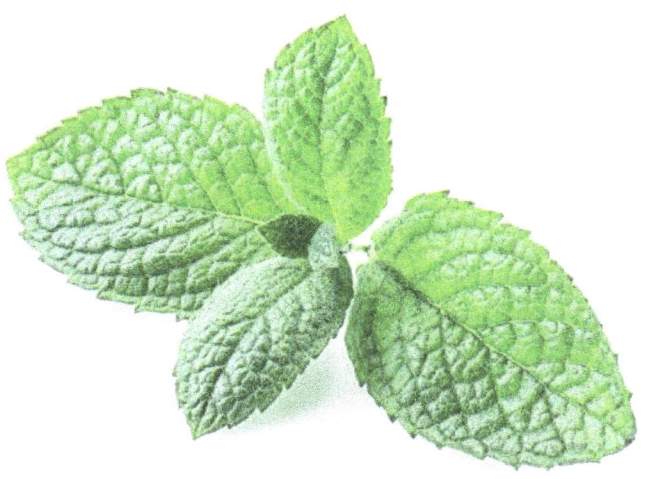

*Picture by Volff*

Leaves from mint plants were mentioned in texts from early Egyptian, Greek, and Roman cultures. They were used as a spice and to scent bathwater and body products and to treat digestive issues. Unlike the ancient roots of other herbs mentioned, peppermint was created in England in 1696 by combining two existing mint plants, water mint and spearmint. It was brought to America with some of the earliest settlers as a favorite flavoring and to treat stomach upsets.

Peppermint is still used to treat irritable bowel syndrome and to relax abdominal muscles, as well as for headaches, fever, colds, coughs, colic, hives, flu, sore throat, and to cool rashes.

Whenever I get a headache, I put a dab of peppermint oil on my forehead. When my daughter was first having burning in her legs after she became ill, I mixed peppermint oil with castor or almond oil and rubbed it on her legs to cool them when the erythromelalgia was unbearable.

You can use peppermint oil on your body with a carrying oil like castor or almond or try a drop or two in your tea. The leaves can be boiled for a refreshing tea or made into throat soothing lozenges. Chopped peppermint leaves make a cool topping for a bowl of homemade fruit sorbet.

# Quinoa

*"Quinoa: The gluten-free grain of the
gods." Bhupendra Chand*

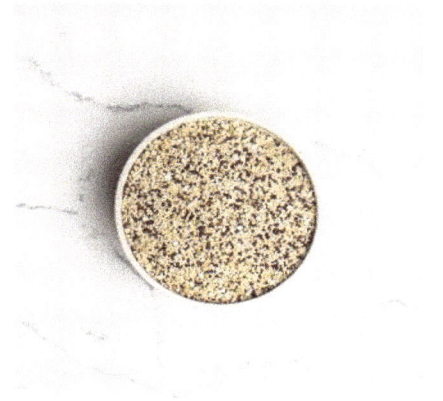

*Picture by Brandi Price*

Quinoa, pronounced "keen-wah," has a rich history in South America and is an ancient grain. It sustained the Incas of Bolivia, Chile, and Peru for more than 5,000 years. They deemed it "the mother of all grains" and it was so treasured that the legends say that the people hosted a ceremony every year during planting season and the emperor planted the first seeds.

This super food was almost destroyed in 1532 by the Spanish in an attempt to wipe out the Incan culture by burning down the quinoa fields. In the Andes Mountains, a small number of crops survived and quinoa traveled out of the mountains in the 1970s and quickly spread around the world as a household staple.

People mistake quinoa for a grain or cereal because it shares the same type of texture and nutrition, but it's actually in the same plant family as spinach and sugar beets, called the goosefoot family. It's not a grain. It's a seed. The leaves of the plant can be eaten just like spinach, but the seeds are prepared similarly to grains.

The United Nations calls quinoa a "super crop" due to its nutritional values and its ability to grown in subpar soil without irrigation or fertilizer. It grows similarly to a weed and can be 3 to 9 feet tall when fully grown with seeds that appear in a variety of colors, though the leaves are more uniform in color.

Quinoa is gluten-free and is considered a super food. It's a great source of plant-based protein with 8.14 grams per cup. Since it offers a variety of amino acids, it also contains lysine, which is needed to synthesize proteins, so this makes it a perfect source of protein for vegans. It also contains more fiber than other grains with 5.18 grams per cup, which aides digestion and helps to keep the colon clear so it's good for constipation and can reduce the risk of diverticulosis, high blood pressure, and high cholesterol.

Quinoa is rich in antioxidants, vitamin E, manganese, iron, folate, magnesium, and quercetin and kaempferol, which are plant compounds that are said to help with protection against diabetes, infections, heart disease, and some cancers.

Quinoa is a staple in my kitchen and we use it at breakfast, lunch, and dinner. It cooks quickly after a rinse just like rice with one part quinoa to two parts water and boil until tender.

For breakfast, you can make it into a cereal and add your favorite nuts and fruits or a plant-based yogurt. For lunch and dinner, add it to patties, tacos, salads, Buddha bowls, and soups and stews.

## Sage

*"How can a man die who has sage in his garden?" Charlemagne era Arabian proverb*

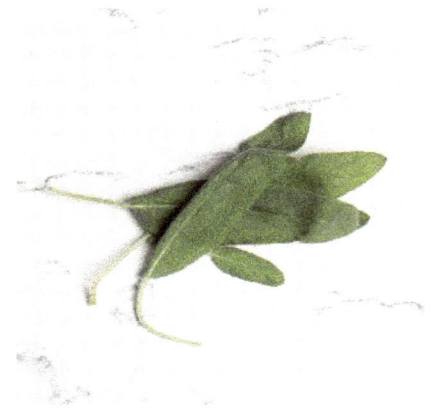

*Picture by Brandi Price*

Sage is originally from the Mediterranean and was called "salvia," meaning to be healed or to have good health and a long life. John Evelyn wrote in 1699 in *Aceteria,* "'Tis a plant, indeed, with so many and wonderful properties as that the assiduous use of it is said to render men immortal."

This plant creates a perfect culinary partnership with fatty foods, so it's often associated with Thanksgiving turkey or pork dishes and it's often ignored the remaining 11 months out of the year. In my family, ground sage is the star flavoring agent for Grandma's homemade stuffing recipe, though I've updated it to make it plant-based. I also like to use sage in pasta dough, savory bread recipes, directly milled into fresh grains, in risotto and butternut squash puree, and when caramelizing onions to add flavor to any dish.

When working with fresh sage, chop it finely and add it at the ending stages of cooking or as a garnish, unless caramelizing onions or sautéing kale or spinach. As you've learned, dried herbs need time to soften during the cooking process and sage will lose its flavor as well as its healing properties as it cooks. If possible, use fresh sage.

Sage is used by herbalists to treat bronchitis, colds, cough, memory, excessive sweating, and a sore throat.

# Seeds

*"The tiny seed knew that in order to
grow, it needed to be dropped in dirt,
covered with darkness, and struggle to
reach the light." Sandra Kring*

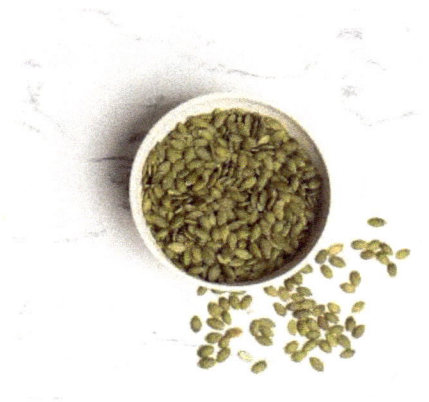

*Picture by Brandi Price*

There are a variety of healthy seeds that can be a delicious and healthy addition to most any meal or snack. It's difficult to pick my favorite one, so for the purpose of this book I'll discuss the two I use most often, pumpkin seeds and cashews.

Pumpkins were first discovered in North America and the seeds have been dated back to 7,000 B.C. in Mexico. In America, as early as 1863 they were listed as an antiparasitic and used as a health aide to eliminate parasitic worms and intestinal parasites.

Today, pumpkin seeds are suggested as a good source for magnesium and help to maintain healthy bones and provide a good night's sleep, nutrients that help to counter the onset of type 2 diabetes, zinc, and can aide in sexual dysfunction by improving urinary disorders and prostate health. Studies that were conducted in Egypt concluded that pumpkin seeds are also an aphrodisiac.

I love to eat plain pumpkin seeds as a snack! They're also a delicious addition to any salad or as a soup topping to add texture and crunch, making a blended soup more filling and satisfying.

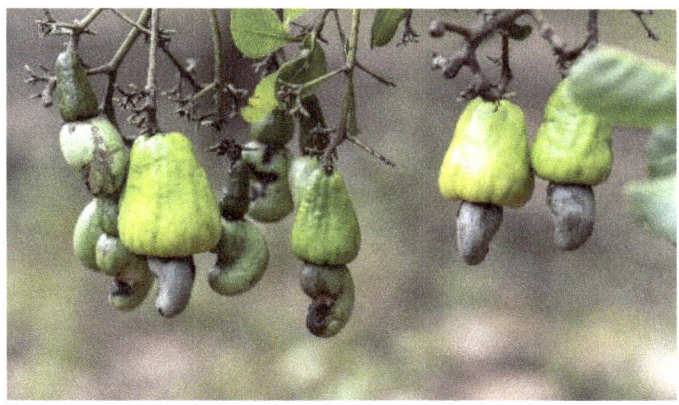

*Picture by Huythoai – Cashew seeds on trees*

Though cashews are referred to as nuts, they're actually seeds!

They grow on trees like nuts and are attached to a large fruit. The seed is protected by two outer shells that are made up of compounds similar to poison ivy and poison sumac. These shells are toxic to humans and must be removed carefully by burning. Even the smoke from burning the shells can be harmful if inhaled, so it's not recommended to attempt to remove cashews from their shells if you're not properly trained. The shells are so toxic that a resin from their shells is used as an insecticide and to make plastics. This is why cashews are one of the most expensive seed options and they're never sold in their shells. Though sold as raw, the cashews are cooked to remove the toxins. No cashew is technically "raw."

Cashews are native to Brazil and in the late 16th century were transported by missionaries to East Africa and India where they have become a staple in traditional recipes.

Cashews are packed with protein, nutrients, and vitamins, including antioxidants, copper, healthy fat, fiber, iron, magnesium, manganese, phosphorus, selenium, thiamine, vitamins k and b6, and zinc.

My family eats cashews almost every day. They're the star ingredient in my daughter's breakfast pudding. I blend them and add an acid and seasoning to make sour cream. They're the base for all my white sauces for pastas and other dishes. And I grab a handful to eat as a healthy snack in the late afternoon when the snack bug hits. I love them!

# Sweet Potatoes

*A sweet potato "comforts, strengthens, and nourishes the body." John Gerard*

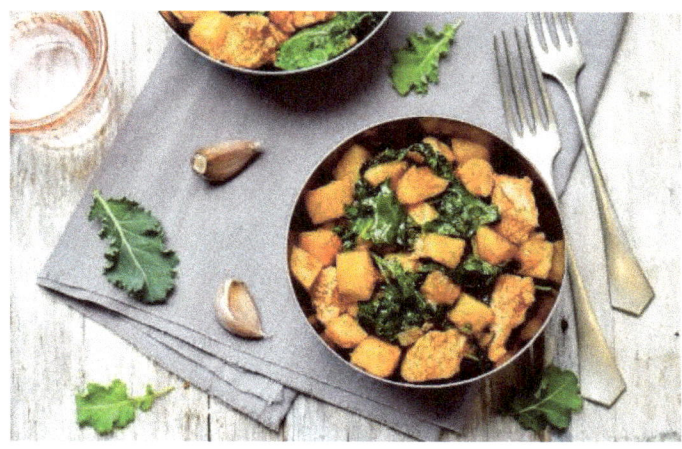

*Picture by Nata Vkusidey*

Sweet potatoes originated in South America and they were used as a primary food source in South America for at least 5,000 years, yet archeologists have discovered proof that they were in Polynesia from 1,000 to 1,100 A.D. with several possibilities on how that occurred, including Polynesians traveling to South America earlier than proven or the seeds hitching a ride across the ocean on seaweed or in a bird's wings. In Central America, sweet potatoes were grown in what is modern day Virginia by 1648. At some point after 1740, the term "sweet" was added to the name to distinguish it from the Irish or white potato.[93]

Sweet potatoes contain both soluble and insoluble fiber. Soluble fiber breaks down in water and basically flushes out of your system. Insoluble doesn't break down in water, so they're not digestible, and they remain in the digestive system to aide in gut health.

Your gut is a host to millions of bacteria. When you feed the good bacteria, your digestive system will operate properly and it strengthens your immune system. A low fiber diet starves the good bacteria. With nothing to live on, the bacteria eats the mucus lining in your gut, which allows the bad bacteria to grow and your immune system to go into overdrive, trying to counter the effects of the bad bacteria on your entire system. This leads to inflammation and illness. Sweet potatoes help to provide good gut bacteria.

They're also rich in copper, fat, manganese, niacin, pantothenic acid, potassium, protein, and vitamins A, B6, and C.

These potatoes are versatile and can be popped into the microwave and cooked quickly for a fast lunch or baked wrapped in foil. We like to eat sweet potato fries that I either bake or cook in the air fryer or you can cut it into cubes and roast for a savory addition to soups or to puree and add to rice or a risotto. Of course, there is always the traditional thanksgiving option, baked with nuts, fruits, and a sweetener, such as maple syrup.

# Thyme

*"I know a place where the wild thyme blows, where oxlips and the nodding violet grows."* William Shakespeare

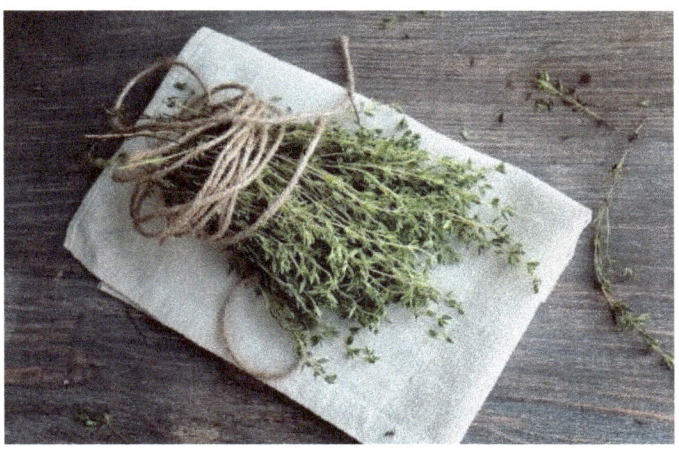

*Picture by Studio Dagdagaz*

The name comes from the Greek word, "thymon," meaning strong odor. The use of thyme for medicinal purposes dates to both the Greeks and Romans, but even the Egyptians used thyme in their embalming process, believing the flowers on the plant would help the departed souls to rest.

Thyme is a hardy herb and is best prepared by adding to the beginning of the cooking process. I like to keep a prepared mixture of dried thyme, rosemary, and oregano on hand for adding to pasta or savory dishes. Using a mortar and pestle, I grind the three herbs together and keep the mixture in a small glass jar for use in cooking. For a finer grind, you can use a coffee grinder. My daughter enjoys fresh thyme in a cashew sauce for another layer of flavor. Try adding thyme to a noodle or rice vegetable soup when you're experiencing cold or flu symptoms and it will open up your sinuses and help you to breathe.

Thyme is so effective that Hippocrates used it is his remedies. Today, it's used to treat asthma, bronchitis, colds, coughs, digestion, flu, for fumigation, and to control high blood pressure.

# Turmeric

*"I am a Hindu because of*
*sculptured cones of red kumkum powder*
*and baskets of yellow turmeric nuggets,*
*because of garlands of flowers and*
*pieces of broken coconut, because of the*
*clanging of bells to announce one's*
*arrival to God, because of the whine of*
*the reedy nadaswaram and the beating*
*of drums, because of the patter of bare*
*feet against stone floors down dark*
*corridors pierced by shafts of sunlight,*
*because of the fragrance of incense,*
*because of flames of arati lamps circling*
*in the darkness, because of bhajans*
*being sweetly sung, because of elephants*
*standing around to bless, because of*
*colourful murals telling colourful*
*stories, because of foreheads carrying,*
*variously signified, the same word -*
*faith." Yann Martel, "Life of Pi"*

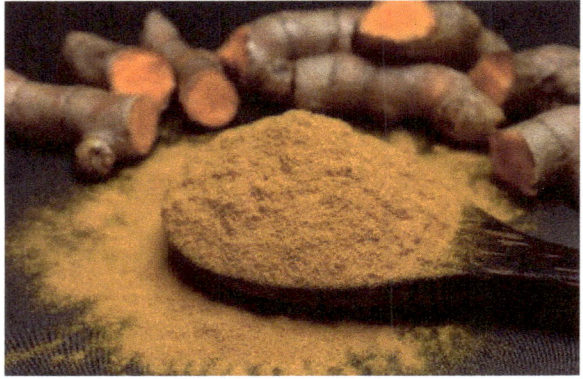

*Picture by Natthapol*

Turmeric was mentioned in the first texts known to Hinduism as a plant that signified purity. It is not only used widely in Indian cooking, but is also rooted in the culture and even used during wedding ceremonies. Turmeric has a long history in Asian communities as well as in medicine. Its use in the United States was much later as people recognize its successes as a natural anti-inflammatory.

Though turmeric is best known as an anti-inflammatory, it's used today as a treatment for issues with the liver and skin, such as eczema. It helps to reduce cholesterol and cancer patients have shown in trials that it helps with oxidative status after radiation or chemotherapy. It also works well as an anti-diarrheal and for Crohn's and ulcerative colitis.

In my kitchen, we drink turmeric in teas, and we also use it as a spice or base for traditional curries.

# A WHOLE FOODS PLANT-BASED DIET CAN ALLEVIATE CHRONIC ILLNESSES

*"Each of us has a unique part to play in the healing of the world." Marianne Williamson*

In 1953, Dr. Roy Swank published a book entitled *Treatment of multiple sclerosis with low-fat diet*. The book has been so well-received in treating multiple sclerosis (M.S.) that it was updated multiple times with the last publication in 1987. Dr. Swank's premise came about in the 1940s when he surmised that people who lived in areas where fish was the main source of protein had fewer instances of multiple sclerosis than their meat-eating counterparts. Using this hypothesis, he weighed the amount of fat content in the different proteins and prescribed a low-fat diet to his patients suffering from M.S. and reported positive changes.[94] In 1990, Dr. Swank summarized 34 years of experience tracking the low-fat diet method of treatment and reported that the 144 patients who stuck with the diet of less than 20 grams of fat intake per day experienced less severity and progression of symptoms and a lower mortality rate with a 95% survival rate than those who ate more than the prescribed amount of fat.[95]

Researchers wanted to put Dr. Swank's claims to the test and chose 61 multiple sclerosis patients to participate by placing 29 in a control group and 32 on a low-fat diet, taking scheduled blood draws and MRIs to test their progress and having the diet group adhere to a low-fat plant-based diet consisting of no meat, fish, eggs, or dairy products and less than 10% fat, 14% protein, and 76% carbohydrates. While there was no measurable difference in large MRI scans or M.S. relapses after one year between the two groups, the diet group reported having less fatigue, lower total cholesterol, a lower body mass index, and better control over insulin numbers. The researchers concluded that with a low-fat plant-based diet, the patients would experience better cardiovascular health if they remained on the diet and small improvements in their conditions were noted, but the study was focused on large improvements, so another study would need to be conducted to properly document the noted changes.[96] A whole foods plant-based diet can be used to treat and prevent some conditions, but not all.

## Osteoarthritis

More than 27 million Americans or 20% of adults are diagnosed with osteoarthritis. It is the most prevalent form of arthritis in the nation and is recognized as a malformation that causes both subchondral bone and cartilage to deteriorate, causing pain, stiffness, swelling, locking of joints, and effusions to occur. Clinical options for treatment usually involve medications, lifestyle changes, and even joint replacement as the effects become disabling. Since animal products are high in arachidonic acids and they have been found to increase inflammation, a plant-based diet has been tested on rheumatoid arthritis patients with positive results, so researchers wanted to discover if the same would hold true for those with osteoarthritis. Researchers chose 37 participants to complete a six-week study and put 19 on the whole foods plant-based diet and 18 in a control group where they made no changes in diet. At the end of the study, it was determined that symptoms of osteoarthritis can be alleviated with a plant-based diet as the participants who followed the diet reported more vitality, energy, and less pain.[97]

## Type 2 diabetes

Type 2 diabetes is affected by the fat eaten and the fat worn and a plant-based diet can help to eliminate both issues. Researchers wanted to determine if a plant-based diet could reduce the prevalence of type 2 diabetes and pooled data of 160,188 females from the Nurses' Health Study and Nurses' Health Study 2, and 40,539 males from the Health Professionals Follow-Up Study who reported no chronic illnesses at the time the studies began. To evaluate the data, the researchers gave positive scores to healthy plant foods and negative scores to animal products and unhealthy plant foods, such as white potatoes. Over the course of the study, there were 16,162 diagnoses of type 2 diabetes with the end determination that those who consumed higher fat foods and animal products and those with higher levels of body mass index had a substantially greater risk of developing type 2 diabetes than those who ate low-fat plant foods and maintained average weights.[98] Their data proves that the risk of type 2 diabetes goes up significantly if you eat fat or wear it.

## Mental health in children

A poor diet has been found to have a connection to poor mental health in children. Dietary patterns and mental health evaluations were recorded in 12 studies performed on children ages 4.5 to 18 years and researchers pooled the data to determine if poor dietary habits contributed to mental health issues. Out of the 82,779 children and adolescents, it was determined that those with healthier diets had a better mental attitude than those who consumed food with a low nutritional value. Researchers concluded that since the onset of anxiety issues occurs usually between the ages of 6 and 13, a better-quality diet could alleviate the symptoms and become a viable treatment plan.[99]

## The Mayo Clinic's preferred diet for heart disease, cancer, and diabetes

The Mayo Clinic is a trusted source for health concerns. They provide educational information on rare illnesses and can sometimes find answers when patients are out of options. The Mayo Clinic promotes a vegetarian diet for issues such as heart disease, cancer, and diabetes. According to their website, a vegetarian diet rich in plant-based foods is the best option because it ensures that all the nutrients a body needs to be at its best can be found in a variety of plants.[100] With a leader in healthcare such as the Mayo Clinic promoting a plant-based diet, it should at least be considered as an option.

# DRINK WATER, NOT MILK

*"A drop of water, if it could write out its own history, would explain the universe to us." Lucy Larcom*

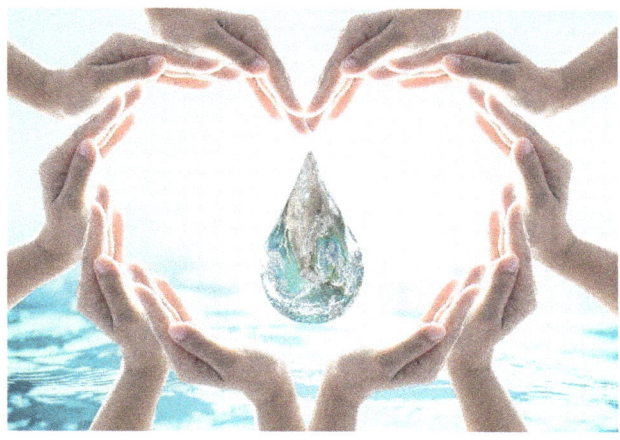

*Picture by Chinnapong*

Whenever scientists are searching for life beyond Earth, they look for life-sustaining water. Wherever water can be found, life is possible.

Within the human body, water accounts for approximately 50 to 75% of our body weight. With that amount of water inside us, it would be feasible to surmise that we could lose water without experiencing adverse effects. However, a loss of 4% of our body's water content could lead to dehydration and, if we lose a mere 15%, we could die. For this reason, I would call water one of the most vital components for human existence.

We need four main elements to live. They are oxygen, hydrogen, nitrogen, and carbon. These elements combined make up approximately 96% of our body mass. The combination of one oxygen molecule and two hydrogen molecules creates H2O, also known as water. Water is a polar molecule, and it bonds best with other polar molecules, such as itself. This bonding aids water in traveling through systems, such as from soil to the roots of a plant, or throughout a human body to provide the ability for the body to function.

A human body can survive for weeks without food, but only three days without water. It's essential as a natural lubricant by aiding in functions such as swallowing and the movement of our joints, and it keeps tissues, such as the eyes and nose, moist. It also softens the waste in our colons to eliminate it more easily and prevent constipation. Chronic constipation is a contributing factor to some cases of colorectal cancer.

Water assists the body in metabolism through thermogenesis, so it's essential for weight maintenance and weight loss. A study was conducted in India in which 50 young females, aged 18 to 23, and overweight with a BMI of 25 to 29.9, were tasked with drinking 500 ml (approximately 17 ounces) of water 30 minutes before each meal, three times per day, over a period of eight weeks. This was an overall increase of 1.5 litres (50 ounces) over their normal daily water intake. At the end of the study, all subjects lowered their BMI or body mass index from an average of 26.7002 to 26.1224, lost weight from an average of 65.86 kgs or 145 lbs to 64.42 kgs or 142 lbs, and their body composition reduced by an average of one inch in their triceps, abdomens, and thighs.[101]

Similar studies provided the same results. In 2003, a study was published in *The Journal of Clinical Endocrinology and Metabolism* which reported that drinking 500 ml of water increases the metabolic rate in males and females by 30%, starting 10 minutes after drinking the water and peaking at 30 to 40 minutes after drinking and lasting for over an hour. In 2011, a study on overweight children confirmed the effect of drinking water and it raised their metabolic rate by 25% and lasted for more than 40 minutes. The conclusions of researchers and scientists involved in these studies were that water increases blood pressure, changes physiology, increases energy available for the body to use and activates the sympathetic nervous system, increases the rate of metabolism by taking fat stored in the body and creating energy from it, and it depresses the appetite.[102]

Water is also an important component of blood, and it helps with circulatory functions, such as transferring vital nutrients to organs and eliminating waste. It also helps to maintain a normal body temperature through sweat, which cools the body down, as well as cellular homeostasis or keeping your cells healthy.[103]

Dehydration is detrimental to your health for all the above listed reasons, but it can also cause asthmatic symptoms, which can be alleviated by drinking water because water is necessary for breathing and proper lung function since the lungs consist of 85% water.

I believe that I've proven my point on the importance of water. If you get bored drinking only plain water, add organic flavors to it, such as wedges from a lemon, lime, orange, or pieces of your favorite fruit. I also like plain tea with no sweeteners. Packaged fruit drink powders are considered processed foods and contain sugar and other unhealthy ingredients. Sodas are also unhealthy and diet sodas are even worse. Google the words "aspartame and embalming fluid" and you'll get the idea of why I would never consider drinking a diet soda. Just keep it simple and drink water or healthy variations of flavored water as mentioned above.

To avoid dehydration, there are several methods to calculate how much water you should drink. A simple calculation for water intake is to divide your weight in pounds by 2.2. Then multiply that number by your age and divide the sum by 28.3. The final number is in ounces, so divide that number by 8 to figure out how many cups of water you should drink per day.

For example, a 150-pound, 25-year old person would calculate water intake as follows – 150/2.2 = 68.18 * 25 = 1,704.5/28.3 = 60.23/8 = 8.5 cups of water per day. The older you are and the more you weigh, the higher the number. That's why seniors often struggle with dehydration. They're not drinking enough water.

A 200-pound 50-year old person would calculate as follows – 200/2.2 = 90.91 * 50 = 4,545.5/28.3 = 160.62/8 = 20. If you currently don't drink much water, that sounds like a lot of water, but once you start drinking it regularly and drink it instead of sodas or sugar-filled juices, it won't seem as overwhelming.

You can also just drink half your body weight in ounces of water.

A good rule of thumb to follow is to drink a minimum of 8 to 10 cups of water per day and increase your intake based on your personal needs. If you currently drink one cup of water or less per day, it's unreasonable to expect you to increase your water intake to 8 cups by tomorrow. It could cause other issues. My suggestion would be to increase your intake of water slowly and build up to your ideal amount of water over a period of a few weeks.

My recommendation is to consult your healthcare professional who can take into consideration your age, weight, the level of activity in your lifestyle, your climate, and any other underlying issues that could help to determine the ideal amount of water you should drink. The Mayo Clinic offers this simple guideline by suggesting that men drink a minimum of 15.5 cups of water per day and women drink a minimum of 11.5 cups.

If you're going to exercise or do physical activity where you anticipate water loss through perspiration, prepare in advance by drinking two to three cups of water before exercising to keep from getting dehydrated.

Also, as mentioned, water increases your blood pressure, so I would suggest to stop drinking water for at least 30 minutes before checking your blood pressure if high blood pressure is an issue. Again, if you have any questions, please consult with your doctor.

**Don't drink milk**

While water is essential to human existence, milk is not. Have you ever taken a moment to consider the fact that humans are the only species that drink milk past infancy and *from another species*? Doesn't that make you wonder why we do it and why we think it's normal?

Biologically, cows were not created to provide milk for humans. In fact, studies have shown that milk has adverse effects on the human body. Hippocrates, born in 460 B.C.E., found that cow's milk could cause stomach issues and skin rashes. Yet, throughout history, somehow that information was lost and humans continued to drink it. If we were created to drink milk, why are 75% of African Americans, 100% of Vietnamese, and almost 100% of all Asians lactose intolerant? Half of the Native American population reports being unable to digest milk. Our bodies are trying to tell us something. Are we listening?

American doctors and scientists didn't report the presence of adverse reactions from drinking cow's milk until the early 1900s. Why was this information not shared with the public and passed down through generations? The only information about cow's milk that is widely shared are warnings for new mothers. Every new mother is told by their doctor not to give cow's milk to infants under the age of one. They're told that it's dangerous. Doctors warn that cow's milk does not contain the amount of iron essential for human babies to grow and it can cause blood loss in the intestines of the infant. The high amounts of calcium and casein in milk block the infant from absorbing the necessary amount of nonheme iron and the excess amounts of protein could lead to kidney damage.

Though it's commonly known that cow's milk should not be given to infants, we're led to believe that milk is necessary once the child grows past infancy and turns one year old. We're told that we should consume milk daily for

118

the rest of our lives and that it's necessary for human development. It's amazing to me that we follow blindly in those beliefs without posing the hypothesis that if it's bad for babies, why isn't it bad for us all?

Our bodies develop a digestive enzyme called lactase that helps us to break down lactose. We stop making lactase at around age four. Still, we continue to drink milk. Why?

It's easy to advise someone to cut dairy out of their diets. It's not so simple to find dairy-free foods. Sadly, milk can be found in several processed foods that you wouldn't think would contain milk. The next time you're in a grocery store, turn the package to the nutrition label and ingredients and, at the bottom, you should see a statement that says, "Contains:...." or "Warning" and the common allergen will be listed, such as milk, dairy, or eggs. Sometimes milk is hidden in the list of ingredients, and it can be labeled by several different names.

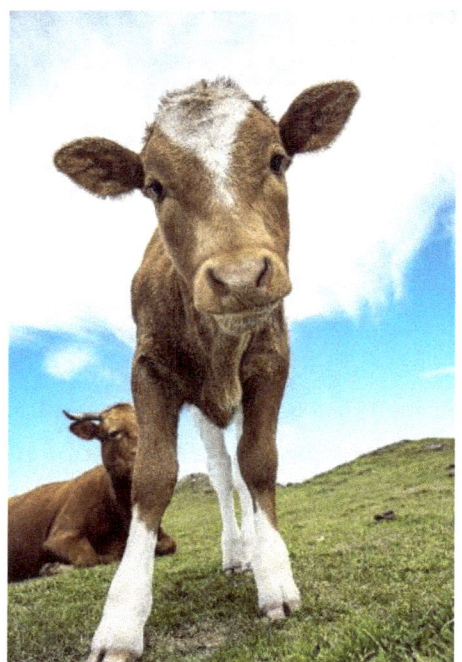

*Picture by Nikokvfrmoto –*

*Milk is for calves, not humans.*

Names for milk on labels.

- o Butter
- o Butter Oil
- o Buttermilk
- o Calcium Caseinate
- o Casein
- o Caseinate
- o Cheese
- o Condensed Milk
- o Cream
- o Demineralized Whey
- o Dry Milk Powder
- o Dry Milk Solids
- o Ghee
- o Lactalbumin
- o Lactose
- o Lactulose
- o Low-fat Milk
- o Magnesium Caseinate
- o Milk
- o Milk Derivative
- o Milk Fat
- o Milk Powder
- o Milk Protein
- o Natural Butter Flavor
- o Nonfat Milk
- o Pudding
- o Skim Milk
- o Whey
- o Whey Powder
- o Whipped Cream
- o Whole Milk
- o Yogurt
- o Zinc Caseinate

And several more names

When we learned that my daughter has a dairy issue, which I explain in detail later in this chapter, we were shocked at how many processed foods contain dairy. At the time of our discovery, the gluten-free craze just started and food companies stepped up and provided several gluten-free options, but almost no dairy-free options could be found in our local stores. At the time, we didn't have a Whole Foods and the few Sprouts and Natural Grocers that popped up in the last few years were several miles from our home. Shopping became frustrating as I searched for convenience foods for my daughter. In those days, the standard American diet or SAD was how we ate, and it became challenging with her dietary restrictions, which also includes a soy issue.

On my daughter's birthday this year, I bought a cake from Whole Foods that I was told was vegan, but I forgot to ask if it had soy. She enjoyed the cake, and her stomach was sick all night. The next morning, she was dizzy. She sat down on her bed in our rented beach house and projectile vomited everywhere; all over the comforter, her suitcase, the carpeted floor, herself. Have you seen the movie *Pitch Perfect*? Of course you have. Then you get the picture. It took hours to clean up the mess and I was reminded to always check the label. The cake contained soy milk. I didn't even bother to check after hearing, "It's vegan." I was excited to find a vegan cake since I couldn't make a cake for her while we were on vacation.

There is a restaurant in downtown Oklahoma City that has delicious vegan comfort food. It's not plant-based, but it's delicious. It's called The Loaded Bowl, if you're ever in Oklahoma. I was so excited when I discovered them, and I couldn't wait to try everything to have an option on days when I didn't feel like cooking since there were no other vegan options in my area. However, when I tried to order food, I learned that almost everything they serve contains soy. Even the deserts. On the occasion when we order food from there, they must make a special dish for my daughter and she's always disappointed in what she gets because she can eat it at home. It's nothing new. Just some mashed potatoes and vegetables.

This is just a reminder that even vegan restaurants don't always serve food that everyone can eat and unless the restaurant is 100% plant-based, always check the ingredients and the labels when ordering or purchasing food. You'll notice that none of my recipes in this book contain tofu, edamame, or soy. Now you know why.

Now back to the topic of dairy, something else that makes my daughter very sick.

The following is just a short list of processed foods and other items that typically contain dairy:

- Bakery items such as cakes, breads, donuts, etc.
- Biscuits
- Breath Mints
- Cake Mixes
- Candy
- Caramel
- Cereal
- Chocolate
- Coffee Creamer
- Cookies
- Crackers
- Granola and Cereal Bars
- Gravy
- Hot Chocolate Mix
- Pancakes
- Pepto Bismol
- Potato Chips
- Salad Dressing
- Sherbet
- Soup in a can or box
- Soy or other Meat Substitutes
- Soy Cheese
- And so on

When we first discovered that my daughter kept getting sick after eating dairy, we had to find a better way to eat! And we did. We cut out most processed foods. Over the years, I've seen new vegetarians or vegans rely heavily on processed foods such as pasta and fake meat or cheese products to recreate the meals that they grew up eating. I understand the appeal. If you're accustomed to eating foods such as hamburgers, hot dogs, tacos, chicken, or spaghetti with meatballs or meat sauce, it seems as if you're restricting your diet too much to not at least replace the foods with imitations. However, in most cases, these foods are extremely unhealthy and since we don't eat soy products and we're still healthy, they're unnecessary to maintain a healthy diet.

To recreate the animal products, companies load them with ridiculous amounts of oil and "natural" ingredients. When you see the word "natural," it doesn't mean healthy or organic. It could be literally anything. Whenever I see the word "natural" on a package, I cringe before placing it back on the shelf. What's more disappointing is the package will usually have the words "plant-based" proudly displayed on the front, tricking the consumer into thinking it's healthy. It's not.

Companies trying to get into the plant-based market are using that term loosely. For example, look at Panera Bread's plant-based options. As of the time of this writing in May of 2021, among other dairy-rich options, they offer Summer Corn Chowder with dairy, Creamy Tomato Soup with dairy, Four Cheese Flatbread Pizza with dairy and white flour and probably with oil, Mac & Cheese, Broccoli Cheddar Mac & Cheese, and even their Mediterranean Veggie has to be ordered without feta cheese. This is a company that is

125

advertising plant-based, but only one item on their plant-based menu could likely fit the description and that's their Ten Vegetable Soup. On the list of ingredients, it doesn't mention what's in their vegetable broth. Often packaged broths are made with oil. If their broth is oil-free, it's the only actual plant-based option on their "plant-based" menu. Are you starting to see how companies trick you? Don't take their word for it. A label pronouncing "plant-based" is likely not as advertised. On a side note, Panera's Ten Vegetable Soup is delicious, and I love their Mediterranean Veggie Sandwich, sans feta.

## Calcium

We're told that animal-based calcium is necessary to maintain healthy bones, yet there is no scientific data to back up that claim. In fact, in countries with the highest calcium consumption, you'll find the highest rates of osteoporosis and bone fractures. In areas that have lower rates of milk consumption, such as the case with farmers in rural communities of Asian countries, they reportedly experience lower rates of osteoporosis, or bone thinning, which leads to bone fractures.

A Harvard study that covered a period of 12 years and involved 78,000 women concluded that those who drank the highest amount of milk, three times per day, were at a greater risk of bone fractures than those who drank little or no milk. In 1994, a study that was conducted on senior men and women in Sydney, Australia, had the same results, with higher dairy intake resulting in higher bone fracture incidents; the risk of hip fractures doubled.[104]

What is often misunderstood is the fact that, in most cases, in developed countries where malnutrition isn't an issue, osteoporosis is caused by calcium *loss*, not calcium *deficiency*.

A healthy diet contains enough calcium to avoid deficiency. So, efforts should be made to maintain the calcium that is consumed and to absorb it properly, not to over-supplement calcium which can lead to other issues. It's really a mindset of use it or lose it. This term is paramount for maintaining good health. In this context, I'm advising that you use the calcium your body is absorbing or your body will lose it.

Stay with me while I break it down and simplify the process.

Calcium is vital in not only maintaining bone and teeth health, with approximately 99% of the body's total calcium stored in bones, but it's also necessary in the areas where the remaining 1% is used. These areas include normal functions of muscles and nerves, blood clotting, and heart health. If this extra 1% is depleted, the parathyroid hormone causes the bones to leak calcium and it goes straight into the bloodstream. Kidneys release calcium into the urine at the same time it's leaked from the bones, and when enough calcium is in the blood, the kidneys release the excess into the urine. This process is how calcium is lost.

Remember that my daughter had calcium in her blood before she became sick. RSD pulls calcium from the bones and teeth. Now that she's recovering, we're spending thousands on dental work. I'm praying that her bones remain strong.

*How do you maintain calcium?*

Calcium is replaced in the body through eating foods that contain calcium or by taking a supplement if the proper nutrition is not available. When replaced with food or supplements, the calcium that was leaked from the bones to help with bodily functions isn't necessarily absorbed back into the bones. This means that ingesting more calcium won't resolve the issue and could contribute to osteoporosis. You can increase your calcium intake, but that doesn't mean your body will cooperate and replace the calcium in areas where it's needed. Your body doesn't run on a computer where you can copy and paste supplements to the places where they're lacking and you can't push a button to fix it. All you can do is take in the right amount of calcium in your daily meals and use the calcium by staying active. Don't over-supplement. Talk to your doctor to find out how much calcium your body needs. We're all different.

The recommended daily allowance of calcium is 1,000 mg for adult women under 50, 1,200 mg for women over 50, 1,000 mg for men under 70, and 1,200 mg for men over 70. Again, taking calcium supplements when you're already eating a calcium rich diet is unnecessary and possibly harmful, unless suggested by your health care professional.

## Where do you get calcium if you're not drinking milk and eating cheese?

Calcium can be found in foods such as fruits, vegetables, nuts, and legumes, which are staples in a plant-based whole food diet. Don't be fooled. The amount of calcium on a nutrition label isn't a measure of how much calcium you'll receive by consuming that product. Calcium is difficult to break down in the gut and only a portion of it will be absorbed into your system. The amount of absorption is called its bioavailability. A simple definition is that bioavailability determines how much of the calcium will enter your circulation system once it's introduced into your body. Bioavailability determines how much calcium your body will be able to absorb. It determines how much will become active and it's a surprisingly small amount, given the high rates of calcium you're accustomed to seeing on labels.

While products such as milk have a higher rate of calcium, its bioavailability is less than that of plant foods, so the amount of calcium absorbed is actually less than calcium found in some plant foods with lower reported rates of calcium. Is your mind blown yet?

Here's an example. One cup of bok choy has 160 mg of calcium and a bioavailability rate of 50%, meaning that 80 mg will be absorbed. Broccoli has a bioavailability rate of 61% while milk only has 30%.

In one cup of milk, you'll absorb 100 mg of calcium.

In one cup of collard greens, you'll absorb 107 mg of calcium.

Getting the picture? You don't need to consume milk to get your recommended daily allowance of calcium.

When consuming calcium from dairy products, it's the same process as other nutrients, such as protein and iron. The cow absorbs calcium, iron, protein, and so on when it eats plant foods. When you eat meat or drink milk, the cow is the middleman in the scenario and the nutrients are first broken down inside the cow and then passed on to you. Why not cut out the middleman and get your nutrients straight from the plant? With so much variety in plant foods available today, we don't need to rely on animals to deliver the nutrition we're lacking, other than B12, which was previously covered and can be supplemented.

Keep in mind that there are some plant foods such as spinach that contain anti-nutrients that bind to calcium and lower their bioavailability. If you want to increase your calcium intake, avoid anti-nutrient foods during meals that include high bioavailability foods.

Foods high in oxylates that bind to calcium and inhibit absorption include beans, beets, berries, cranberries, some dark green vegetables such as spinach, as well as nuts. Beans, seeds, and nuts are high in phytic acid, which also binds to nutrients such as calcium and prevents absorption.

Following is a list of foods that offer high bioavailability and therefore increase intake of nutrients such as calcium. Enjoy these foods as a snack by themselves or combine them with brown rice or quinoa for a meal.

| Plant Food | Calcium | Calcium Absorption % |
|---|---|---|
| Broccoli (1 cup, boiled) | 62 | 61 |
| Brussels Sprouts (8 sprouts) | 60 | 63.8 |
| Collard Greens (1 cup, boiled) | 268 | 40 |
| Kale | 94 | 40.9 |
| Mustard Greens (1 cup, boiled) | 165 | 57.8 |

| | | |
|---|---|---|
| Orange Juice, calcium fortified (1 cup) | 349 | 37 |
| Plant milk | 350 | 30 |
| Tofu, calcium set (1/2 cup) | 861 | 30 |
| | | |
| Source: U.S. Department of Agriculture, Agricultural Research Service, 2011. USDA National Nutrient Database for Standard Reference, Release 26. | | |

For better bone health, instead of over-supplementing with calcium, add more plant protein to your diet and ensure you're getting enough sodium, magnesium, vitamins D & K, and plenty of exercise. When you're active, your bones will hold onto their calcium and prevent leakage. When you're sedentary, your bones will determine that you don't need that much calcium in your system, and they will allow calcium to leak since it's not being used. Get moving! Do something that is weight-bearing, such as walking, lifting weights, yoga, and so on.

Also, go easy on the salt! Excess salt in your body will cause a greater amount of calcium to be lost through your kidneys. If you're a smoker, consider quitting. You're at a 40% higher risk of bone fracture than non-smokers. Quitting is not only beneficial for your bone health, but also prevents ailments such as heart disease and cancer.

**Milk is unkind**

Milk is so detrimental to our existence and both cruel and deadly to cows that Gourmet magazine's contributing editor,

Anne Mendelson, called it, "The milk of human unkindness." Did you know that the average age of a cow is 20 to 25 years? In the dairy industry, a cow rarely lives to the age of 6. At 2, female cows are impregnated artificially and their babies are taken from them and sent to the slaughter house to be cut up for veal, a "delicacy." Then the mother is hooked to a machine and milked. This pattern is repeated during her productive years, usually capping out when she turns 6. Unproductive milk cows are no longer useful, so they're slaughtered.

Not only is the process of obtaining milk from cows on factory farms unkind, but cow's milk carries blood and mucous, which is cleaned for humans to drink. It also includes opiates similar to morphine and an exorphin called casein, a known carcinogenic for humans that is necessary for growing calves. Casein is made to be addictive so that calves return to their mom to get big and fat and grow up to be healthy cows. The addictive factor is why you find it so difficult to give up cheese. It's addictive for the continuation of the species of cows. Not for humans. And we're consuming it!

Milk is also making us big and fat! We're told the more we drink, the healthier we'll become. That's only a true statement if you're a cow.

For the reasons listed, in my opinion, a poor diet includes dairy. Poor diets are linked to 70% of chronic diseases in America. Poor diets are rich with milk, cheese, yogurt, and other harmful dairy products. The average American, either knowingly or because dairy is snuck into their processed foods, consumes approximately 30 ounces of dairy per day, which equals 600 pounds of dairy per year! 600 pounds!!

Can you imagine what it's doing to your system?

To your brain?

Yes, I said brain.

When my daughter attended public school, she was required to drink milk every day with her lunch. The cafeteria monitor insisted that she finish her carton of milk "to get strong and healthy." She was always a thin child and I suppose they thought she wasn't getting proper nutrition at home, so they insisted that she drink it. After her second year in third grade, she was diagnosed with dyslexia and she had issues concentrating at school. She never liked milk. I would even go so far as to say that she hated it. A few years ago, I read an article by Dr. Manik G. Hiranandani in which he described a link between dyslexia and reactions to dairy products. His story was a mirror image of my daughter's. I have yet to find studies that back up this claim, but the possibility of a connection is intriguing.[105]

Like those monitors in her school cafeteria, I grew up believing that milk was important for a child to flourish and to become strong and healthy. I also pushed milk on her at home, but I can't remember forcing her to drink a glass of it. She often refused to drink it. Though, her favorite foods were cheesecake, fettucine alfredo, and mac and cheese. She ate dairy products, but usually only on special occasions. Looking back, I believe her slender lanky frame came from her digestive issues that began as a newborn. For the first six weeks, I tried breastfeeding her, but she cried constantly, didn't gain much weight, and had diarrhea. Her pediatrician suggested I stop feeding her and to put her on a soy-based milk and it worked. She could digest soy as an infant and she became a healthy happy baby. I wish the doctor would have told me instead not to drink a glass of milk every morning or eat eggs or cheese or all the other stuff I consumed in my efforts to ensure that she was getting the best nutrition. Maybe then I would have figured out there was an issue with her digesting dairy products and eggs and her teachers wouldn't think of her as malnutritioned. Also, I'm not sure how she was able to digest soy as an infant, but not as an adult. It's fascinating how the human body changes and develops.

At every birthday party as a child, she ate fettucine and cake with ice cream and then her friends would bang on the bathroom door and beg her to go out and play, but she was either throwing up or too sick at her stomach. We thought it was nerves and too much excitement. We didn't know that her favorite foods were making her sick.

At the age of 18, she concluded that she had a dairy sensitivity. My husband and I performed blind tests on her to see if it was real or not by sneaking milk, cheese, and eggs into her food. Every time, she would get sick and not just for an hour or for the evening, but for three days. And it wasn't just diarrhea; her heart would race, she'd break into a cold sweat, her head would hurt, and her stomach cramped so much that she didn't feel like eating anything. I guess it's good that we were poor because her favorite rich foods were unaffordable except for special occasions. For breakfast, she liked peanut butter toast. For lunch, she ate a sandwich with a slice of processed cheese and for dinner, she'd eat whatever meat I cooked with canned vegetables on the side. On a normal day, she didn't eat much dairy, so on special occasions, her body would go into shock.

After she figured out the fact that she had an issue with both eggs and dairy, we soon learned about how severe reactions to dairy during a school day can interfere with how the brain functions. At school, she couldn't keep up with the class and had difficulty understanding math and couldn't read on the same level as her classmates. I removed her from school when I was told she needed to repeat third grade and attend special education. After one year at home where she wasn't forced to drink milk and didn't consume dairy products daily, she surpassed her classmates and was tested the following year at the school and was able to read on college level. I'm not sure if it was the absence of dairy being forced on her or the personalized attention that made the difference in her ability to comprehend, but I believe that eliminating the daily jug of milk helped.

## Bottom line: Scientists say that milk can make you sick

By drinking milk, some doctors state that you have a risk of developing what is called Johne's disease in cattle and referred to as Crohn's in humans. A good friend of mine was diagnosed with Crohn's at the age of 19. She has been on disability because of her disease since her early 20s. Her digestion issues control her life. Her diet is limited to foods that aren't stringy and are easy to digest. She can't eat celery, mushrooms, corn, pineapple, seeds, nuts, foods with skin, or salad, and so on. Every six months she undergoes an invasive procedure during which the doctor dilates her colon because she develops strictures in it and food can't pass through easily, making her very ill. Some cases of Crohn's are well managed with medication, and some require the removal of the colon altogether and for a colostomy bag to be used to remove waste.

A group of scientists at the University of Liverpool believes that Mycobacterium paratuberculosis is transferred from cows to humans through dairy products. This bacterium prevents white blood cells from killing E.coli, which is found in Crohn's patients in higher than average numbers.

Professor Jon Rhodes explains that "Mycobacterium paratuberculosis has been found within Crohn's disease tissue but there has been much controversy concerning its role in the disease. We have now shown that these Mycobacteria release a complex molecule containing a sugar, called mannose. This molecule prevents a type of white blood cell called macrophages, from killing internalised E.coli." Previous to this finding, it was discovered that Crohn's patients have a weakened defense against E.coli and larger numbers of a specific kind of E.coli that is "sticky." The professor's next reported step is to find out if a combination of antibiotics can kill the bacteria and treat Crohn's. [106]

According to my friend with Crohn's, nobody in the Crohn's community with which she has ever communicated can digest milk and they avoid it. She has never been able to digest milk from her earliest memories, like my daughter. Therefore, stating that she developed Crohn's from drinking milk like the scientists in Liverpool have hypothesized is not an accurate statement, but it's interesting. Could the connection be from earlier generations or have occurred in infancy? Who knows?

Crohn's is a disease that has just recently gained enough traction to begin studies on its cause and possible cures. It will be interesting to see what the ultimate conclusion of the connection between Crohn's and milk will be, or if there is a connection.

## Conclusion

I could write an entire book on the reasons why milk is bad for the human body and how my daughter and I gave up dairy years ago and are still alive; no health issues from not drinking milk. But this book isn't titled *Milk is Evil*, though I might write that book someday. It's about plants and how they heal your body.

Bottom line? Drink water, not milk.

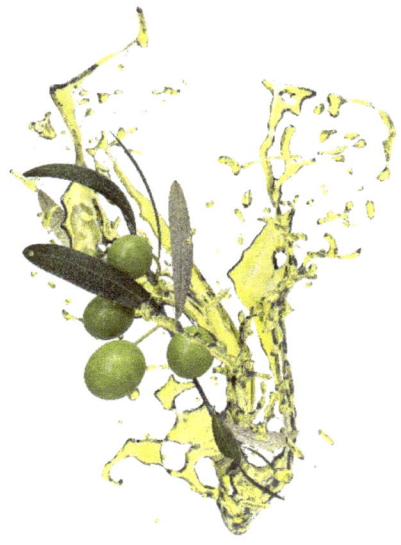

*Picture by Giovanni Cancemi*

# OIL IS NOT A HEALTHY FAT

## Macro- and Micro- nutrients

*"No oil is healthy!" Jody Ortiz*

Your body requires macronutrients to function properly. Macro means large, so these are the largest amount of nutrients your body needs. Macronutrients provide the most energy and are vital to your existence. They are protein, fat, and carbohydrates. All of these are a necessary part of your diet. You can consume them in an unhealthy way, by eating meat, oil, and white rice, or you can choose the healthy alternative and get them from eating plants. As I've expressed numerous times, you don't need animal products as a source of macronutrients. You can find them in nature.

Micro means extremely small. Therefore, micronutrients are the smallest nutrients, such as vitamins, and they're also a necessary part of your diet. You ingest these by either eating plants and going straight to the source or supplementing with vitamins and pills. If you're eating a plant-based diet, other than B12, which we already covered, micronutrients are in your food. Unless you have a specific condition that makes your body low in certain vitamins and minerals and your doctor suggests it, there is no need for supplementation.

Both macronutrients and micronutrients are necessary, and unfortunately in the standard American diet, they're overconsumed and come from unhealthy sources. Throughout the pages in this book, I've provided studies and evidence that support this claim. To make sure that you understand macronutrients and the healthiest sources, let's break it down.

**Protein**

Sources of plant-based protein are covered extensively in previous chapters, but since protein is the second largest component in the human body, only second to water, protein is a vital macronutrient and I want you to understand that animals are not the best source. They're the middleman. You get a cleaner, healthier version of protein if you go straight to the plant and cut out the middleman.

To recap, though protein is second only to water in your body, you don't need to consume large amounts of protein to maintain good health. The recommended daily allowance of protein for a 50-year-old female of average height and weight is 58 grams. In the plant world, this is equivalent to eating a breakfast of oats (7 g/cup) and chia seeds (12 g/4 Tbsp), or what's called overnight oats; a kale (2.5 g/cup) salad for lunch topped with pumpkin seeds (7 g/4 Tbsp), carrots (2 g/cup), and cucumbers (1 g/cup); and a lentil (18 g/cup) patty or soup for dinner with mushrooms (5 g/cup) and broccoli (4 g/cup). The total amount of protein you'll consume if you follow this plan is 58.5 grams. On an average day, you'll likely eat a larger variety of plants and add snacks and sides to your meals. If you're eating a variety of plants, you're taking in plenty of protein. There is no need to stress over the amount of protein in your food. Just eat plants.

To figure out exactly how much protein your body needs, multiply 0.8 grams times the kilogram measurement of your weight. If you're a petite 30-year-old female, weighing 125 pounds, that averages out to be 56.7 kilograms. Multiply that number by 0.8 and that's a little over 45 grams of protein.

Here is a simple chart with just a few of the most common plant foods and their protein levels to use as a reference. As you can see, there is protein in the plants that make up a daily healthy diet. Just eat plants.

| Plant | Protein in grams | Plant | Protein in grams |
|---|---|---|---|
| Almonds | 7 grams/4 Tbsp | Flax seeds | 8 grams/4 Tbsp |
| Bell pepper | 1 gram/cup | Hemp seeds | 10 grams/4 Tbsp |
| Black beans | 15 grams/cup | Kale | 2.5 grams/cup |
| Black-eyed peas | 14 grams/cup | Lentils | 18 grams/cup |
| Broccoli | 4 grams/cup | Lettuce | 1 gram/cup leafy or romaine |
| Brown rice | 5 grams/cup | Mushrooms | 5 grams/cup |
| Brussels sprouts | 4 grams/cup | Oats | 7 grams/cup |
| Cabbage | 2 grams/cup | Onion | 2 grams/cup |
| Carrot | 2 grams/cup | Pinto beans | 14 grams/cup |
| Cashews | 4 grams/4 Tbsp | Potato | 5 grams/small white with skin |
| Cauliflower | 2 grams/cup | Pumpkin seeds | 7 grams/4 Tbsp |
| Celery | 1 gram/cup | Quinoa | 5 grams/cup |
| Chickpeas | 15 grams/cup | Sesame seeds | 7 grams/4 Tbsp |
| Chia seeds | 12 grams/4 Tbsp | Spinach | 1 gram/cup |

| Collard greens | 4 grams/cup | Split peas | 16 grams/cup |
|---|---|---|---|
| Cucumber | 1 gram/cup | Squash | 2 grams/cup |
| Green peas | 8 grams/cup | Sunflower seeds | 8 grams/4 Tbsp |
| | | | |

# Fat

### Fat – No oil is healthy!!

A question that comes up often is why don't plant-based vegans consume oil? Coconut and olive oil are healthy, right?

Nope!

Here's why:

Oil is a processed food.

It consists of 100% fat pulled out of a plant.

It's all the bad parts of the plant with no nutrition.

A healthy heart is maintained by a low-fat diet.

Low-fat diets are recommended to treat and prevent diabetes.

If you're eating 100% fat from oil, that's 100% fat, not low-fat.

All oil is the same; be it coconut oil, olive oil, peanut oil, avocado oil…it's oil.

NO OIL IS HEALTHY.

However, your body needs fat. Not bad fat from oil. Good fat.

Good fats on a plant-based diet include whole avocados, whole nuts, whole olives, whole seeds, and even flaxseed. These are whole foods that aren't processed and stripped of fat. When eating them whole, you're also getting fiber to digest them and properly break down the fat.

Three groups of fats:

Simple – A simple fat has the same genetic makeup of sugar or carbohydrates of carbon, hydrogen, and oxygen. Though they're made from the same ingredients (speaking in chef terms), they're denser, like a slice of bread, and they contain more energy than sugar. The most common of this type of fat are triacyl glycerides with a primary function of keeping your skin oily and from drying out and to transport blood and fat to and from your liver.

Compound – These fats are made from a simple fat and compounded with another type of fat to create more fat.

Derived - Once fat is in your body, it's converted into a different type of fat, such as cholesterol. This is a derived fat.

I don't want to get too technical on what happens to fat when it enters your body, but I do want to make it clear that too much fat of any kind overloads your system and makes you sick, causing diseases such as coronary artery disease, type 2 diabetes, and fatty liver disease. How the fat behaves once it enters your body depends on the source of the fat.

## Healthy whole food fats

- Avocado – Can be used in dressings, sauces, dips, toppings, and on sandwiches. An avocado is ripe when it turns dark green, almost black. If it's bright green, it's not ripe. Sit it on a counter until it ripens or if you're not going to eat it for a few days, put it in your refrigerator to slow down the ripening process. If it's black and papery feeling, it's too ripe. An avocado is just ripe when you push in the stem and it easily sinks into the fruit. In my husband's family's kitchen in Mexico, avocados and tomatoes are consumed daily and they remove the seed and place the fruit upside down on the table between meals and then cut off the dark layer on top before serving. You can store a cut avocado in the same way or place it in the refrigerator wrapped in a paper towel with cut side down or drizzle it with lime juice and put it inside a glass bowl or plastic bag. The recommended serving size of an avocado is ¼ of the whole fruit, so if you're eating alone, you'll want to figure out which way you prefer to store the leftovers. While your body needs fat to function properly, too much is detrimental.

- Flaxseed – These are whole seeds that can be ground or purchased ground. They are small enough to incorporate into most recipes without the texture being altered, but they will add a binding agent, so they work best in recipes such as pancakes, muffins, and so on. If you're low on testosterone or hormones, ask your doctor how much flaxseed to consume because it doesn't just bind to food products. It will remove excess hormones and testosterone in your system through your digestive tract. And yeah, it can be a jolt to your digestive system if you're not accustomed to eating it. Small amounts are best. Start with 1 tablespoon per day and never exceed 5 tablespoons in one day. Store flaxseed in your refrigerator or freezer to keep it fresh.

- Olives – My daughter loves olives. I don't. They're too bitter for me. She eats them on pizza or in Greek salads or pastas and in wraps. You can also eat them with a snack plate of celery and hummus. The recommended serving size of olives is 5 to 10 whole olives. Once opened, olives need to be stored in the refrigerator in an airtight container.

- Nuts – Since I don't like olives and my digestive system isn't a fan of avocados or flaxseed since having e-coli and c-diff and no gallbladder since age 19, my digestive system is sensitive, so I eat nuts and seeds to get my necessary intake of fat. I use nuts on salads and in muffins and I snack on a couple of raw almonds throughout the day. I also enjoy toasted nuts mixed with maple syrup and balsamic vinegar on roasted brussels sprouts and as salad dressings. Serving sizes on nuts differs, depending on the type of nut. I would suggest no more than 10 nuts per day. Almonds can be stored at room temperature in an airtight container, but soft nuts such as walnuts and pecans must be stored in the refrigerator to keep them from molding. Have you ever tasted a moldy nut? I have. Don't make the same mistake. Store your nuts properly.

- Seeds – I buy small quantities of seeds and use them quickly, so I store these in an airtight container in the cabinet, but if you buy a large bag or eat them slowly, it's best to store them in the refrigerator. Seeds such as cashews, however, are already cooked so I keep those in the cabinet. Cashews are the base for my bechamel sauce, sour cream, and Italian salad dressings. I also use them to thicken recipes and in pudding. I use sunflower and pumpkin seeds as salad toppings and on quinoa or cacao balls. Seeds can be used in a variety of recipes or toasted and stored as a topping. The standard serving size of seeds is one ounce, which is approximately 4 tablespoons when considering a seed the size of sunflower seeds.

**Coronary artery disease and oil**

Oil saturates most of the fast foods that our teenagers are eating. It's on fries and burgers and chicken strips. It's even in those "plant-based" burger patties that are touted as a healthy alternative to meat. Oil is so prevalent in our food that according to Dr. Esselstyn, leading expert in healing CAD with plant-based foods, our country's high school graduates receive their diploma along with the start of coronary artery disease by the time they're 18![107]

Dr. Esselstyn explains that when you consume oil, your blood cells and endothelium get "sticky." The endothelium is a tissue that lines your blood and lymphatic vessels and heart. When it gets sticky, blood doesn't flow through your veins undisturbed. At this point, your LDL becomes oxidized. The endothelium will request white blood cells to rid it of LDL, which fill up so much that they turn into foam cells.

Remember that by age 18, if you're eating what most teenagers eat in the Western world, you've already developed plaque in your arteries. When the plaque is disturbed, it releases into your blood stream and causes a heart attack. Immediately after eating bacon and eggs or sausage and hashbrowns or a burger and fries, the process of developing sticky blood and endothelium takes place and a foam cell is created. That foam cell glides through your blood vessels, banging into everything in its path, and ruptures the plaque, blocking the artery and triggering a heart attack.

This process occurs after consuming oil…any type of oil. Oil makes your blood and endothelium sticky and it injures your endothelial cells. So does sugar, which we'll get into later.

Your body can't differentiate if the oil was stripped from an olive or used to deep fry a piece of chicken. Oil is oil.

To reverse this process and keep from developing foam cells that disturb the plaque that you've already developed, you'll want to reverse the oxidation process of your LDL by adding nitric oxide into your system. Plaque is made from oxidative inflammation. Antioxidants (nitric oxide) counter this process.

When I first quit eating meat, I went to Whole Foods and walked into their vitamin and supplement area. I explained to the employee that I quit eating meat and I wanted to know what supplements I needed to take. Like you, I was concerned about missing important nutrients in my diet. I thought I needed to eat animals to survive, so I must need to take supplements to make up for what I was no longer eating.

The very helpful gentleman working that day knew exactly what I needed, and the main supplement he suggested was L-Arginine. This supplement boosts nitric oxide, but it also can lead to death if you have a history of heart attacks and cause issues such as gout, nausea, bloating, worsening asthma, and so on. I didn't take it after reading about the side effects, especially since I have asthma, and I wouldn't suggest it for you, unless your doctor says it's safe to take. This is just another example of taking a pill when you can get what you need from nature. I'm not sure why he equated me eating healthier to needing a pill that opens arteries, but the important and only supplement I needed was B12, and that wasn't even on his must-have list. I didn't learn about the importance of B12 for almost a year after quitting meat when I developed neurological issues and saw a neurologist. Her son was vegan, so she knew right away exactly what I was missing – B12.

Aside from unnecessary supplements with harmful side effects, nitric oxide, or antioxidants, when consumed through diet, keep your blood flowing, arteries dilated, and prevent high blood pressure and plaque buildup. How do you add nitric oxide to your system without supplementation? Just eat plants.

Green leafy vegetables are antioxidants.

Dr. Esselstyn suggests eating a handful of green leafy vegetables 6 times per day for 3 to 6 months to get you started, and then continue to eat green leafy vegetables every day for life. This is especially important as you age because your body will slow down on the process of converting food into nitric oxide.

Green leafy vegetables are kale, spinach, swiss chard, collard greens, brussels sprouts, cabbage, asparagus, and so on. Cook these vegetables for at least 5 minutes and add them to your meal as side dishes or toppings, but do not believe that you will get the same benefit from them if you put them into a smoothie. Chew them! This helps to convert them into nitrates, and you don't want the added sugar of fruit, which we all love in smoothies. Instead, as Dr. Esselstyn says, "Chew your greens!"

In my recipes and in the chapter titled "Chef secrets," you'll find techniques to cook foods without adding oil. It's possible and once you really taste the food without saturating everything in oil, which coats the ingredients of your dish and doesn't allow sauces or seasonings to stick, diluting the flavors, you'll fall in love with the tastes of real food.

## Carbohydrates

I've already explained how low-carb diets can be detrimental to your digestive system, but as a macronutrient, you can surmise that carbohydrates are a necessary part of your daily diet. In fact, the Dietary Guidelines for Americans recommends that 45 to 55% of your daily diet should consist of carbs. This is a short list of the plants that contain the complex carbs your body needs.

- Fruits
- Grains
- Legumes
- Nuts
- Seeds
- Vegetables

Basically, if you're following a healthy plant-based diet, you're getting your recommended daily intake of carbohydrates. Let's discuss the healthy choices, which don't include white rice, processed and bleached flour, or sugar.

**Whole rice and grains**

Rice is the seed of a semi-aquatic plant. It comes in varieties and is differentiated by color, whether it's long or short grain, and its texture – sticky or fluffy.

Rice is whole when it contains the bran, germ, and endosperm. This whole grain is called brown rice. It's the most nutritious and filling with a chewy texture and nutty flavor. The cooking process is also much longer than white rice because of the difference in texture as it is a whole grain.

As described in chapter four, when rice is processed, it's put through a mill to remove the bran and germ, leaving only the endosperm. The final product is white rice. All the nutrition is removed, leaving just a starch with no fat or fiber. It's turned into pure sugar, which is not a complex carb and is not on the recommended list for your daily intake of carbs.

Grains are the edible seeds of grass plants, and like rice, contain a germ, bran, and endosperm, and some have an outer shell or husk. Once the husk is removed, the whole grain is revealed. The bran is the outer layer, and it contains fiber and flavor. The germ is inside the bran. It's where the grain stores its fat. The endosperm is the soft inside and is the largest part of the seed. The whole grain provides nutrients and fiber. If it does not consist of all three parts of the whole grain, it's no longer nutritious.

Cut or cracked grains are still whole, as none of their nutritional layers are removed. Yet, their cooking times are shortened, and their texture is altered when the grain is cut, such as in whole wheat flour.

If a grain has been processed, such as in pearled barley or white flour, it's no longer considered a whole grain and it doesn't hold the same nutritional value. Therefore, it's not a whole food and not a component of a healthy plant-based diet.

## Sugar

Like casein, sugar is addictive. It can alter your mood and make you feel happy when you're on a "sugar high," and when you crash as your blood sugar reacts to the effects on your system, you'll crave it again and the cycle continues. Too much sugar can lead to obesity, low energy, and headaches. The extra sugar in your body turns into fat, which leads to heart disease and other health issues.

Sugar that comes in a complex form is recommended for a plant-based diet, meaning from a whole fruit with fiber. In chef school, I learned how to make fruit pastes to use as a supplement for sugar, which is how I came up with the idea to use medjool dates for sugar in my recipe for my daughter's cacao cashew pudding. You've probably heard that some chefs use applesauce in pasta and cakes as a binding agent, which is also a healthier way to eat sugar.

Another reason to avoid sugar is that most white sugar is processed using bone char, which is the bone of cattle, to filter it into the white color. Brown and confectioner's sugar are created from additives to white sugar, so they're also likely to contain bone char, unless you find a certified vegan brand. These are simple sugars and they're not broken down in your body like complex carbs, so even the vegan brands are not considered healthy or plant-based. In my kitchen, I use either fruit, fruit pastes, or turbinado or coconut sugar.

# THE ENVIRONMENT

*"I don't want you to be hopeful. I want you to panic." Greta Thunberg*

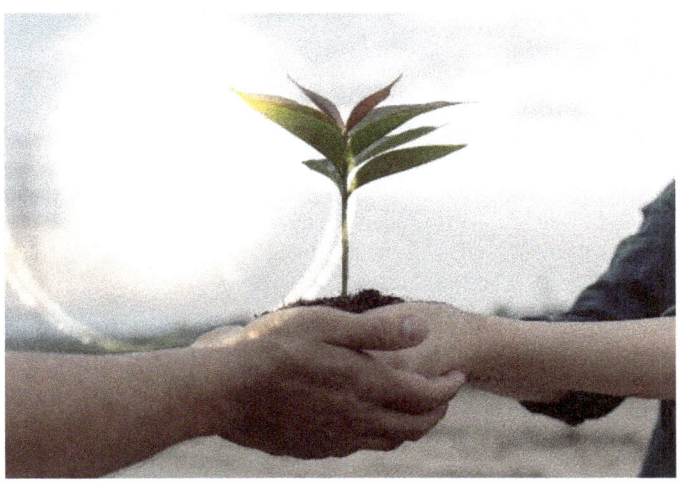

*Picture by Puwasit Inyavileart*

It's no secret that the meat and dairy industries use a lot of resources when caring for livestock and clearing land for the purpose of grazing cattle. This practice is only adding to environmental issues.

Researchers wanted to study different dietary patterns to determine which diet would be the most sustainable and help to feed underdeveloped countries, thus eliminating diseases caused from starvation while healing the land. They found that eight times more land is required to sustain an omnivorous diet versus one that is vegan.

In this study, ten diets were put to the test and measured based on the current USDA's reports of food consumed within the United States. The diets included categories such as omnivores, ovo-vegetarians, pescatarians, and vegans. Researchers concluded that to feed an omnivore following a healthy diet plan, 1.08 ha's are needed per person per year. In measurements, a ha is a hectare and 2.47 acres equals 1 hectare. Vegans, on the other hand, only need 0.13 ha's per year. In land equivalency, omnivores require a lot more land to eat than vegans, meaning vegans leave the smallest footprint in terms of land consumption. Therefore, more people could be sustained with a smaller amount of land and resources if everyone followed a vegan diet at least a few days per week.

## Biodiversity: Cultivating sustainable living on planet earth

With the current toxic status of our planet, it's possible to create a sustainable plan that will impact not only our generation, but generations to come, and allow for healthy air, water, and food to continue to be natural resources for our environment.

According to World Population Balance's website, Earth's current resources can only sustain two billion people based on a current European standard of living. However, our planet is populated by seven billion humans, and the population is growing. This means that we're currently using more than double the amount of our resources with no recovery time in between. Our planet does not have time to recover the loss from our over-consumption. Even the poorest countries — who consume only a fraction of the number of resources as industrialized countries — are using their resources at a rate of over 10% of what they have available.[108]

Imagine that you have a glass of water sitting in front of you with a replenishment rate of two ounces per hour. The water is being replenished, so it may as well be used. You stick a straw into the glass and drink over six ounces per hour. At that rate, the glass will eventually be emptied because the rate of use is going faster than the rate of replenishment. Though it will eventually be refilled, you could suffer from dehydration while waiting for more water if you're drinking at a higher than sustainable rate. This is what happens when resources are used faster than they are created. This is what we are doing to the earth. Sadly, in the process of depleting the natural resources, we're also polluting them, so that the rate of replenishment will eventually stop altogether, or the life-sustaining resources will become too toxic for our systems. It's imperative that changes are made that will impact our environment before it's too late. Changes made, just one person at a time, can have a ripple effect. Mahatma Gandhi said, "Be the change you want to see in the world." Change starts with us.

If we don't change our environmentally devastating practices, to maintain our current rate of growth without suffering losses to starvation or malnutrition, going green in not only our lifestyles, but also our diets, may be the answer. Our planet is rich with nutritional foods that grow naturally and without any growth hormones or antibiotics that are often given to livestock and poultry by factory farms.

Our "green" foods have been around for millions of years, and they have sustained numerous species. Though studies show that human beings became smarter and stronger once we introduced high protein foods into our diet, the world is now much smaller when considering supply chains and available resources. High protein foods such as seeds, nuts, legumes, and even many of the plants can be found at local farmer's markets or in grocery stores. Therefore, eating meat is now considered an option, and one that in the past few decades has become the choice that most health professionals would call unhealthy.

Additionally, the best way to help the planet and still maintain a healthy diet is by eating local. University of Florida's Living Green program has found that, on average, food travels 1,500 miles from the farm to the table.[109] This means that not only is the food leaving a large carbon footprint as it makes its way to a meal because it's loaded onto semi-trucks that use a lot of diesel and emit pollution into the air, but it also has a high possibility of rotting and wasting during transport. With so many hungry people in the world, it's unthinkable that in an effort to make money, big businesses are letting food go to waste. This is one reason I support programs such as Imperfect Foods. Every week I have groceries delivered that are either overstocked or on the verge of expiring. I save money on groceries, and they're not wasted and thrown away. I also support a local farm that delivers fresher produce than what is available in the stores.

In the past few decades, corporations have turned to the farming industry where they take over small farms and bring in heavy equipment that cause more pollution and ruin the soil. Farmlands that have been owned and maintained by families for generations are going bankrupt or find themselves forced to sell their homes because big business is taking over. By purchasing locally grown food, a local farmer makes an income, which is then distributed back into the area through taxes and everyday living. This promotes other local businesses, and the food is healthier and fresher.

Local farms are also necessary for critters. Outdoor spaces that are filled with food, instead of livestock, ensure that wildlife and insects have a home for the continuation of their species.

## Oh, the meat industry

The meat industry is another area where sustainable living can make a difference. Raising livestock takes up natural resources in grains and water, and they create greenhouse gases.[110] These gases have a devastating impact on the earth's temperature near the surface and have eradicated thousands of miles of homes for wildlife in the areas that are melting due to global warming.[111]

Former ranchers such as Howard Lyman, the "Mad Cowboy" have led the way in changing how we view their industry and people like him have gone on to create sustainable businesses that help the environment instead of harming it. By following this trend, ranchers can provide more space for wildlife and cut down on resources that are used to feed livestock that emit gases.

## Go vegan!

Vegan diets also promote heart health and can help combat diabetes and create a healthy lifestyle. When someone chooses to go vegan, they not only save the animal from the plate, but they save resources and provide habitats for countless other animals. In summary, veganism saves lives, jobs, and creates a stronger community with better resources.

Though I've demonstrated how eating green and going vegan can help save the planet, there will, of course, be challenges to overcome. The biggest challenge is raising awareness to the fact that living green is more than just a slogan. Going green affects not only the environment, but also the economy. The United Nations calls it "sustainable development."[112]

The situation is so vital to our survival, with so many challenges ahead of us, that Switzerland is just one of the countries that is stepping up and trying to set an example for change. Global warming is causing devastating snowfall amounts and ruining roads, wildlife habitats, and tourism in their country.[113] New York City heard the call and planned to spend $2.4 billion in building a green infrastructure to create a sustainable city.[114] I can only imagine how our planet would change if every city in the world made such a valiant effort.

If more communities would become involved in making a change and work toward educating the general population on where our food comes from, how it makes its way to the stores, and what resources are used in the process, we could all make a more educated decision about what we eat. A vegan plant-based lifestyle is the healthiest choice, not only for us, but also for the world around us. Choosing to eat vegan saves lives—including our own.

Many people argue and say that we were made to be carnivores and that our main source of food should come from protein. Most of my friends define protein as meat. My response is that if God intended for us to survive by eating animals, and that was the only way we could live, then He would not have made so many nutritional foods that grow on their own that we're still discovering in sparsely populated regions to this day.

I believe that sustainable living is possible. I believe that education will be key to the survival of our precious resources, as well as our planet. Then, and only then will we become a truly self-sustaining planet.

As a miracle-minded coach, I believe in miracles, and I will continue to hold this belief. We can change. Change begins with us.

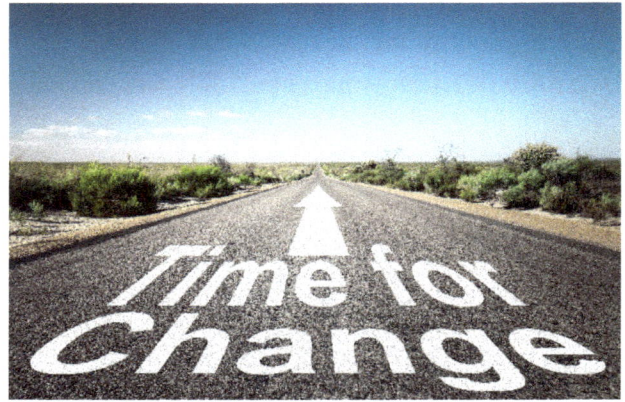

*Picture by Magann*

# SUMMARY AND CONCLUSIONS

*"The measure of intelligence is the ability to change." Albert Einstein*

A vegan plant-based diet provides the nutrition a human body needs to not only survive, but also heal. This was my thesis statement in my college capstone paper, and it still holds true today.

As proven in the research provided, a plant-based vegan diet can help to prevent chronic diseases such as cancer, heart disease, type 2 diabetes, and others, as well as heal the body of chronic illnesses. Too many people follow the standard American diet and have ongoing chronic issues with their health as a result. Diseases such as cancer could become less of a challenge if cancer contributors such as animal-products, high protein diets, and processed food consumption were reduced.

Misinformation provided by historical governmental documentation on nutrition starting at the turn of the 20th century only added to the issues that were destined to arise. In my opinion, organizations such as the American Heart Association, American Cancer Society, and the American Diabetes Association perpetuate misinformation about a healthy diet with promotions of animal-based foods.

Studies centered on switching to a vegan diet have yielded promising results in health issues. Scientists are learning that to heal the body and prevent certain chronic issues from occurring such as cancer, heart disease, and type 2 diabetes, a plant-based vegan diet is the best option, though a plant-based diet is still being studied to be a viable treatment for issues such as multiple sclerosis. To make the change, more education for doctors and nutritionists must be made available and a part of the required curriculum.

The cost of health care in the United States could be greatly affected if more people switched to a plant-based vegan diet. Issues such as heart disease cost services like Medicare and Medicaid millions of dollars per year and it could be avoided.

Mental health is also an issue to be considered when discussing the best diet options for diseases such as cancer because loved ones of cancer patients suffer from more pain, lower levels of financial stability, and higher instances of depression. Poor mental health in children is also a concern when a child is not eating a healthy diet.

Finally, the sustainability for the planet is greatly affected because those who follow a plant-based vegan diet not only leave a smaller footprint as far as the amount of land it takes to feed them, but also more food would be available to feed those who suffer from diseases due to starvation, leaving a better sustainable capacity to expand our population.

By switching to a whole food plant-based vegan diet, people can (a) live longer and healthier; (b) have better mental health, (c) reduce the cost of health care, and (d) help to save Earth and the growing population on the planet for generations to come.

Are you ready to make the switch?

# GOING PLANT-BASED

*"Veganism is not a sacrifice. It is a joy."*

Gary L. Francione

One of the arguments that I hear the most when discussing the possibility of someone switching to plant-based vegan is the expense of eating plants. Unless you're an extreme couponer who lives on mostly processed foods, eating plants is actually more budget friendly than eating meat. Though I haven't eaten a bite of meat since May of 2013, and my attempt at a piece of turkey that Thanksgiving, which I spit out, my husband thinks he needs it to survive. I buy meat and cook it for him. I'm not great at it and I don't enjoy touching it, smelling it cook, or cleaning up afterward so I buy a lot of prepared foods, such as pasta meals or air fried chicken pieces in the freezer section. Occasionally, when there is nothing else to feed him, I cook a boneless skinless chicken breast and a box of mac and cheese. I cook two meals every single night, unless I'm making one of his vegan favorites, such as chickpea patties or a pot of pinto beans.

When we pick up food from his favorite restaurant, Outback Steakhouse, he eats the grilled shrimp, sirloin steak, macaroni and cheese, house salad with ranch dressing, and bread. I order a dry baked potato and steamed vegetables with no butter and I eat a small amount of bread. I'm sure you can guess which meal costs less. I basically eat sides while he eats expensive steak and seafood. You could say I'm a cheap date, which I remind my husband of as he pays the bill. Haha!

Every night I make sandwiches for my husband and his crew with white sandwich bread, onion and tomato slices, mayonnaise, processed sandwich meat, and American cheese product.

He eats a completely different diet than my daughter and I, which includes mostly processed foods and very few vegetables. He's very likely unhealthy on the inside, but he's happy, so I don't push anything on him. He'll change when he's ready. I share this because like me, you may eat meals with someone who won't consider a vegan diet. It's okay. Don't force it. Change occurs eventually and by demonstration, not force.

I say this, though I did force my daughter to switch. That was a different situation. She was bedridden and sick, and I prepared all her meals and wanted her to heal. See the difference?

In the meantime, I buy healthy plant-based foods as well as processed junk food and meat. There is a huge difference in the cost, not just in restaurants. When you make the mental shift from considering what you formerly ate on the side as a main dish, you'll understand how not buying meat, dairy, and all the processed foods will save money over time.

People are under the assumption that if you eat plant-based vegan, everything you eat must be organic. That's not the case.

Have you ever heard of the dirty dozen?

Every year, the Environmental Working Group releases a list of the top 12 dirtiest produce that contain the highest exposure to pesticides. It doesn't matter how much you wash or peel them; they're still going to remain "dirty." These are the items that you want to purchase labeled "organic" or grow them at home, if possible. Everything else you can purchase from conventional sources, unless you choose to eat all organic.

This is the list for 2021, according to EWG. Remember to check the list each year, as it changes.[115]

- Strawberries
- Spinach
- Kale, collard greens, and mustard greens
- Nectarines
- Apples
- Grapes
- Cherries
- Peaches
- Pears
- Bell and hot peppers
- Celery
- Tomatoes

# Food sources

You can find a lot of the pantry foods on Amazon's website. These are the top 25 foods I purchase from Amazon.

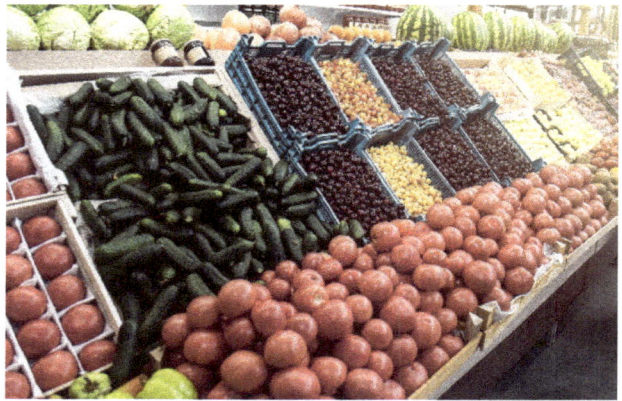

*Picture by Olinchuk*

1. Split peas
2. Chickpeas
3. Lentils
4. Einkorn wheat berries to mill for flour
5. Nutritional Yeast
6. Tea
7. Arrowroot powder
8. Protein powder
9. Brown rice
10. Cashews
11. Dried herbs
12. Yeast
13. Dried figs and other dried fruits
14. Nuts
15. Pinto beans
16. Vegan chocolate
17. Farro
18. Rolled oats
19. Cacao powder & nibs
20. Quinoa
21. Chia seeds
22. Kosher salt
23. Vegan yogurt culture
24. Fresh bananas
25. Black-eyed peas

My local Sam's Club offers a few organic produce choices, and that's where I buy russet potatoes and romaine lettuce. A local farm delivers fresh select produce year-round and, in the summer, I visit the local farmer's market.

I also order weekly from Imperfect Foods. Their selection is food that is overstocked or on the verge of expiring. It helps the community to cut down on food waste. I've been very pleased with their selection and service, though they don't have everything I need. For those items, I find them on Amazon or go to a Sprouts or Whole Foods.

Whether we're eating out or eating at home, our grocery expense for my daughter and I is always much less than what I spend on my husband, and we eat more meals at home, so I buy more items for us. Again, because we eat minimal amounts of processed food and mostly plants and dried items such as legumes and quinoa, it is much more affordable to feed us than it is to feed my husband.

It may seem like a larger expense at first because you'll stock your pantry with new foods that maybe you haven't tried in the past, but once you have all the necessary basics, you'll spend less money long-term.

# MAKING THE SWITCH

*"It takes nothing away from a human to be kind to an animal." Joaquin Phoenix*

Now that you've learned how both my daughter and I healed our bodies by changing what we eat, and you know the science that backs up the fact that going plant-based vegan is the healthy, safe, humane, and earth-friendly choice, are you ready to switch?

Not sure where to begin?

You have a few options.

It's time to analyze what best fits your lifestyle and which option seems the most realistic for you.

1. Dive in! Go full vegan today! Why let another minute pass? Let's do this!

2. Wade in the water by going vegan five days per week for now and slowly transitioning to seven.

3. Dip your toes by switching to vegan three days per week and having animal products on the other four.

There is no right or wrong way to do this. We're all individuals and have our own needs and cravings, so what works for me may not work for you.

If you've received a diagnosis that led you to this book and you're making the switch for health reasons, then you might want to dive in and get started right away. What do you have to lose? But, if you're just interested in maybe trying it out to see what it's like and you're not ready to commit, then dip your toes or wade in at your own pace, like I did.

Possibly you've made up your mind and you want to switch, but you're still contemplating and you're not sure where to start. This chapter will hopefully put you on the right path. If you still want more information, as a certified health coach, I'm available to work with you and guide you through the process. I'm just an email away...jo@sproutedvegan.com.

## Let's get started

These are a few of the questions that I ask new clients in my 12-week plant-based vegan program. I'd like for you to treat these questions as homework and fill in your responses as you would if you were working with me. Your responses will help you to dig deep into your eating preferences, habits, and you'll be able to target exactly what you need to achieve from your daily sustenance.

If you've ever kept a food journal, these questions will be easy, and you'll breeze through this next section. But if you've never really sat down and evaluated what you eat and when you eat it, this may be an eye-opening exercise for you. This is an exercise just for you, so be honest with yourself in these responses.

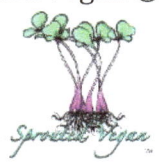

## Sprouted Vegan Intake Form (Partial for book use)

Number of people who share meals with you and will be following your plan.

Adults –

Breakfast _____ Lunch _____ Dinner

_____

Teens –

Breakfast _____ Lunch _____ Dinner

_____

Children –

Breakfast _____ Lunch _____ Dinner

_____

Snacks are shared by how many family members?

_____

### Goals and Readiness:

I am interested in changing how I eat because

_____

_____

_____

_____

_____

_____

_____

_____

_____

_____.

I would like to change these three things about how I eat

1.

_____

2.

_____

3.

_____

I am interested in switching to a vegan diet in this way.
Check which one best applies to you.

_____ Diving in (Going full vegan now Let's
do it!)

_____ Wading in the water (Vegan meals 5
days a week and fish and chicken the other two.)

_____ Dipping my toes (Vegan meals 3 days a
week and fish and chicken the rest of the week.)

My past experience with switching to a vegan lifestyle and why I believe it didn't stick

_____

_____

_____

_____

_____

_____

_____

_____

_____

_____.

## Food Prep and Cooking

I do not eat the following foods because of cultural or religious reasons.

_____

_____

_____

_____.

I have this much time for meal prep/cooking

Breakfast

_____

Lunch

_____

Dinner

_____

Snacks

_____


I need to eat this meal on the go

Breakfast

_____

Lunch

_____

Dinner

_____

Snacks

_____

In my household,

_____

prepares most or all of the meals.

I require guidance from you in the following area in food prep or cooking.

_____

_____

_____

_____


In my household, _____
shops for food.

I eat the following meals and snacks at home

_____
_____
_____
_____.

I sometimes skip the following meals

_____.

I currently eat _____% whole food,
_____% processed food,
_____% fast food.

I currently drink approximately _____ ounces
of water per day.

My primary source of liquid on an average day is

_____.

My biggest nutritional challenge is

_____
_____
_____
_____
_____
_____.

My greatest nutritional brag is

_____

_____

_____

_____

_____

_____.

## Food Intake:

Please respond with a number of servings under the frequency in which you choose the following foods.

| Item | Daily | Weekly | Monthly | Occasionally | Never |
|---|---|---|---|---|---|
| Example: Fruits | 2 | | | | |
| Fruits | | | | | |
| Vegetables | | | | | |
| Legumes | | | | | |
| Nuts | | | | | |
| Grains | | | | | |
| Fermented foods | | | | | |
| Meal replacements | | | | | |
| Desserts | | | | | |
| Snacks | | | | | |
| Home-cooked fresh meals | | | | | |
| Leftovers | | | | | |
| Frozen meals | | | | | |
| Fast food | | | | | |
| Restaurant food | | | | | |
| Cafeteria food | | | | | |

| Vending machine food | | | | | |
|---|---|---|---|---|---|
| | | | | | |

Please use this space to elaborate on types of fast food, vending machine, meal replacement, or frozen meals you eat and why.

_____
_____
_____
_____
_____
_____
_____.

I crave these foods

_____
_____
_____
_____
_____.

I do not want to eat these foods

_____
_____
_____
_____
_____
_____
_____.

Use this space for anything else you want to share that would be relevant to creating a meal plan to best suit your lifestyle.

_____

_____

_____

_____

_____

_____

_____

_____

_____

_____

_____

_____.

Did you have any "aha!" moments? Are you eating healthier than you realized? Or could your daily diet use some work?

My 12-week plan can get you on track to a healthy plant-based vegan lifestyle. Email me when you're ready or make an appointment at www.SproutedVegan.com.

# CHEF SECRETS

*"Being a chef never seems like a job. It becomes a true passion." Gordon Ramsay*

## Chef's tools

This is my list of must-have tools in my kitchen to be able to prepare healthy and nutritious meals. You may not need everything on the list, depending on how often you cook and if you don't enjoy certain cuisines, but these are what I use most often.

- Baking dish – The size you need will depend on how much you want to bake at a time. I have both square and rectangular glass pans and I use them all.

- Colander – You can also use strainer clips or snap strainers. My daughter bought a set for me one Christmas and I don't know how I survived without them.

- Cookie sheet or roasting pan – You'll use this for multiple dishes, but mostly when roasting vegetables.

- Cutting board – Years ago at a craft show, I bought a piece of stone made into a cutting board and it stays out on my kitchen island all the time since I cut something every day. It's easy to clean and I don't need to find a place to store it.

- Dough scraper – These are very handy and can be used to pick up your cuttings from the cutting board and moved to a pan or bowl.

- Food processor – Surprisingly, I don't use mine very often. I added it to the list in case you don't have a high-speed blender or if you're physically unable to mash chickpeas and lentils. I can mash food quickly with a pastry cutter and my blender works on a lot of dishes, but some people need extra help. This is probably my least used tool, but it does come in handy when making salsa. I don't use it because I don't enjoy cleaning it.

- High-speed blender – Get a Vitamix or Blendtec. I tried a Ninja and returned it the next day. It didn't work on my cashew sauces or smoothies. There were chunks of cashews and other stuff such as almonds for my potato soup that it couldn't handle. If you can't afford a good high-speed blender, then use a food processor and save up for a blender.

- Knives – Invest in good knives. A dull knife can cut you just as easily as a sharp knife because dull knives have to be maneuvered through the food and they can easily slip and cut you while a sharp knife cuts straight through with less maneuvering.

- Knife sharpening steel – After every use with your knife, to keep it sharp and in good working order, wash it with warm soapy water, rinse, dry, and pull it over a knife sharpening steel at a 45-degree angle on both sides a couple of times. You don't need a fancy knife sharpener.

- Pastry cutter/Dough blender – I use this tool to mash beans and chickpeas when I don't feel like getting out the food processor and cleaning it. And I use it for pastry.

- Pots & pans – At least one pot that will hold soups and stocks plus one large and one small sauté pan. I bought a stainless steel Wolfgang Puck set eight years ago at Sam's Club for $99 and it works perfectly for most of my cooking needs. I also have one set that is nonstick that I use when making pancakes and chickpea patties.

- Salad spinner – If you dry your greens after washing, which you should always do, drying them right away will keep them from wilting. You definitely need a salad spinner. Also, a metal bowl with a lid to store your greens.

- Utensils – I use wooden spoons, silicone spatulas, and tongs most often.

- Vegetable peeler – Invest in a good one. I like Pampered Chef or Cuisinart.

## Batch cooking

The best advice I can give to you on saving time in the kitchen is to cook the foods you eat often, such as roasted vegetables, lentils, chickpeas, quinoa, and butternut squash puree and sautéed kale in batches. You can use these ingredients in multiple recipes throughout the week and it makes prepping for meals much faster.

Use the quinoa and roasted vegetables and legumes to build a quick Buddha bowl (a bowl with quinoa and veggies) and use butternut squash puree as a base for soup, pasta sauce, or "cheese" sauce.

The roasted vegetables will stay good for three or four days after cooling and placing them into an airtight container and storing them in the refrigerator. Sometimes I eat them for up to a week, but never past one week. Store cooked quinoa in the same way. It will keep for up to a maximum of five days. No longer. The butternut squash puree will stay good up to five days. Lentils and legumes will keep for four days.

To help you keep track of how long the food has been stored in the refrigerator, either place labels on the containers with the date they were prepared or cook them on the same day each week. That's how I batch cook. I receive my order from Imperfect Foods on Monday, so I batch cook on that day. I know that I need to eat everything by Thursday or Friday, depending on what it is.

Another note, I don't use plastic, except as lids for glass bowls. Invest in a good set, such as Pyrex or other reliable brands because glass can be placed in the bottom rack of the dishwasher and is the most food safe alternative, plus it doesn't add a plastic, refrigerator taste to your stored food. My city has a glass recycling container that is always open to recycle glass. I avoid plastic whenever possible.

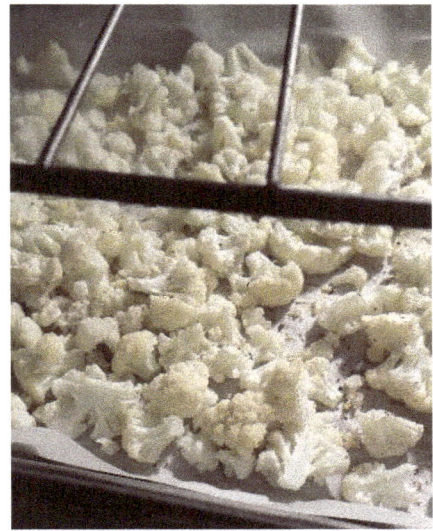

Batch cooking roasted cauliflower.

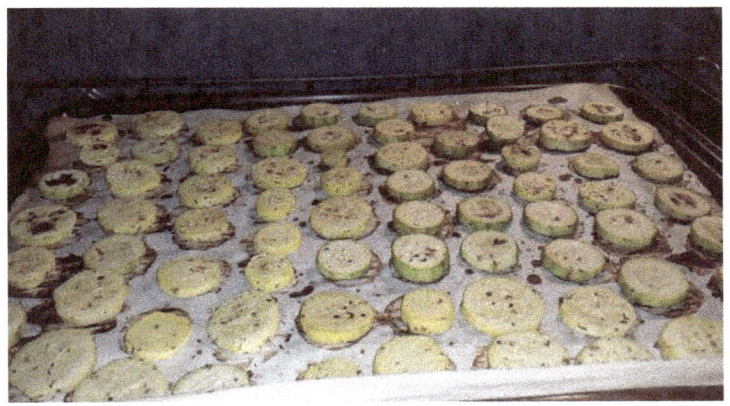

Batch cooking yellow squash and zucchini.

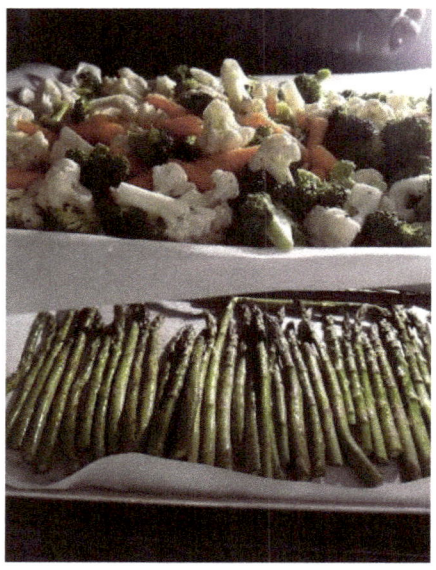

Batch cooking mixed vegetables and asparagus.

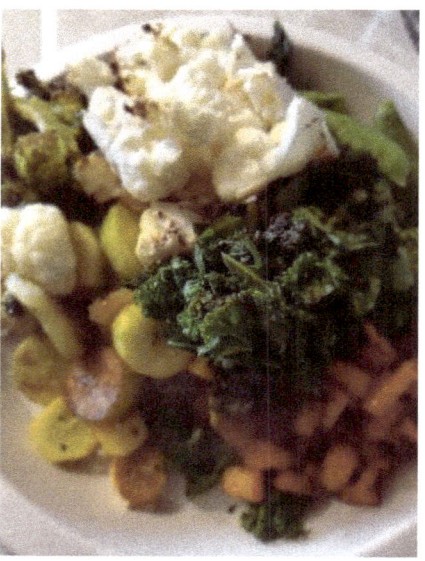

Quick Buddha bowl made from batch cooking.

## Storing lettuce

I've tried several ways to store lettuce and make it stay fresh and crisp. The best option I've found is to wash it right away, spin it dry, and store it in a metal bowl with a lid. Romaine lettuce stays fresh for up to three weeks in my metal bowl. You can also make your salad ahead by preparing the cabbage, lettuce, and carrots and storing it in a metal bowl. However, wait to add soft ingredients such as cucumbers and peppers when it's ready to serve because they will get mushy and wilt the rest of your salad.

Also, I shouldn't need to mention this, but I realize that someone reading this may be new to cooking. Never ever pre-dress your salad. Always add your dressing just before serving.

When eating salad or any type of cold food with something hot such as quinoa, always put the hot item on the bottom of the dish and stack cold items on top. The steam from the hot item will wilt anything cold underneath it and make it mushy. I allow the hot item to cool for five minutes before adding cold items on top.

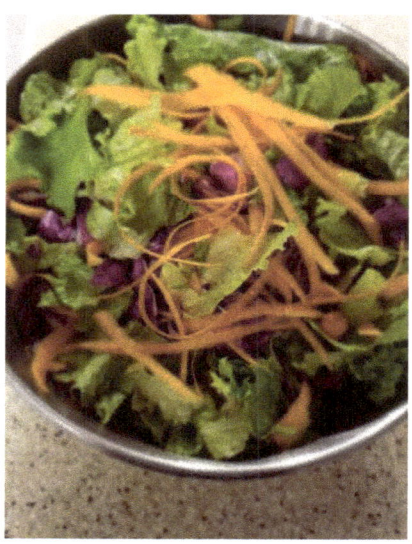

## Cooking with herbs

When cooking with herbs, add the dried herbs to the dish at the beginning process of cooking. This will allow the herbs to soften and add flavor to the dish. If you wait to put them in at the end of cooking, they will disrupt the texture of the food and the dish won't have the amount of flavor you desire.

Fresh herbs are added either at the time of plating a dish or at the very end of cooking – within the last five minutes. When adding the herbs, first rinse them and then cut or rub them between your fingers to release their full flavors. Depending on the herb, I use the stem as well as the leaves, such as with cilantro, a family favorite. The stem isn't too hard and it also carries wonderful flavor. However, with herbs such as rosemary, the stem is hard and unless I'm grinding the herb, which is unnecessary for fresh herbs, I don't use those stems.

When storing fresh herbs such as cilantro and parsley, place them stem side down in a cup of water, like you would fresh flowers, and place a plastic bag over the top and store them in the refrigerator. This creates a greenhouse effect (the good kind, not the bad) and will allow the stems to continue to live and feed on the water, making them remain fresh for a longer period of time. The following picture shows cilantro purchased on the same day from the same package with one stored properly as described above. See how the cilantro just left in the package is wilted, but the cilantro stored in water and covered is still fresh? You can use any one-gallon plastic bag or grab a plastic produce bag from the produce section at the store and use it.

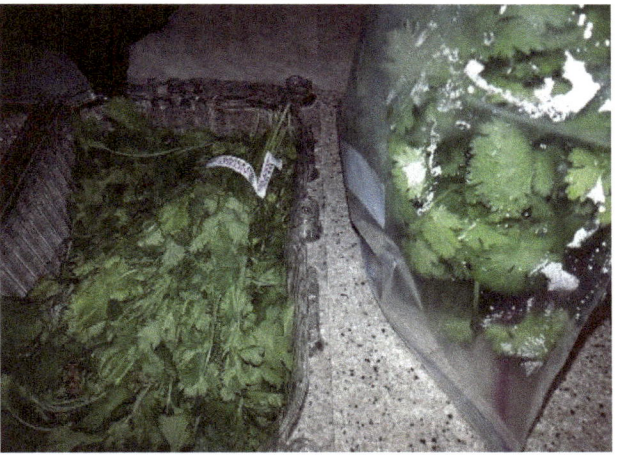

Cilantro stored in a cup of water and covered in plastic vs cilantro left in the package.

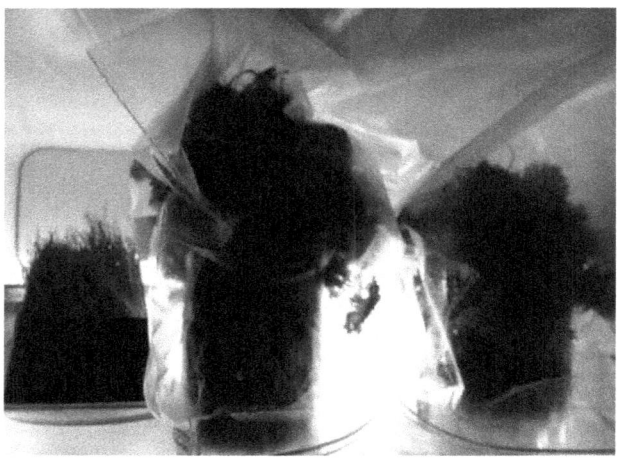

A greenhouse in the refrigerator.

**Pasta**

I enjoy making homemade pasta. My mom once told me that the happiest she ever saw me was when she sat in the living room and watched me crank out the pasta on the metal pasta roller. I was sweaty and working hard, but I was smiling. I was in my element.

My homemade pasta on the
drying rack.

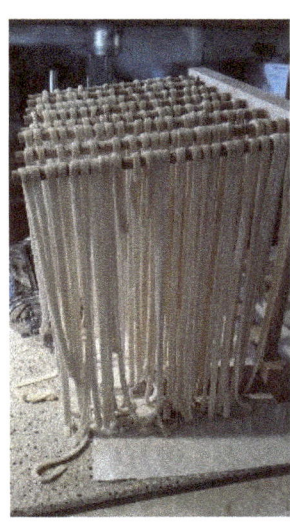

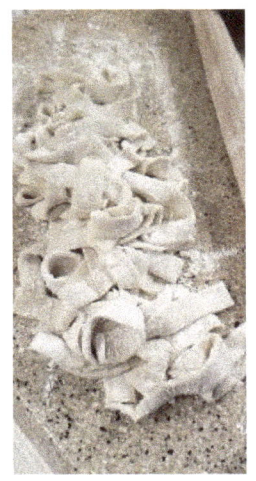

Making fresh udon noodles.

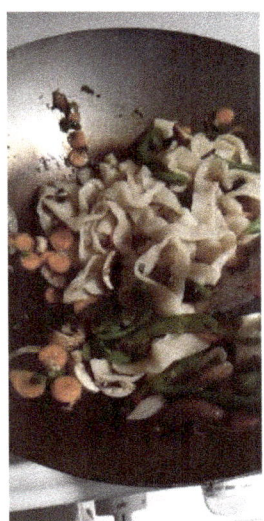

Cooking a stir fry in the wok with freshly made
udon noodles.

Unfortunately, I don't always have the time to make fresh pasta, so when I get the craving for it, I look at the package labels and choose a pasta that is made with whole wheat or rice flour, and of course, no dairy or eggs. I've tried the chickpea and buckwheat pasta, but I didn't like the texture as well and the flavor of the sauce didn't hold up to the pasta. It disappeared, no matter how many herbs I added.

Cooking pasta is the same technique, whether fresh or dried. Bring your pot of water to a boil and add salt after the boiling starts. Make sure that the pot is large enough and that it is filled at least halfway with water so that the pasta can move around freely, not stick together, and cook evenly. DON'T ADD OIL!

Instead, make sure that your water is boiling when the pasta hits the pot, stir it occasionally so that it doesn't stick, and rinse it with cold water immediately after it's drained. While draining the pasta, reserve one to two cups of the pasta water in a heat safe bowl or cup. This reserve can be added to the blender if you're making a bechamel (white sauce) to clean out what sticks in the blender to get all the sauce for your pasta, or added back into the pasta when mixing in the sauce. This step aids the sauce in attaching to the pasta and will allow the flavors to develop in your final dish.

## Roasting vegetables

I love roasted vegetables! They're so delicious and filling and they make a great addition to several types of recipes.

To roast really tasty vegetables, I suggest the following:

- o Preheat your oven to 425. That's the temperature I use on all roasted vegetables, though some cook for different lengths of time.
- o Line a large cookie sheet or roasting pan with parchment paper. By using parchment paper, you'll have no need for oil. They won't stick to the pan and you can just add the paper to your compost, wipe the pan clean, and you're finished with your cleanup.
- o Wash and cut all vegetables to the same approximate size. The size you use doesn't really matter. You can roast half a cauliflower head to make cauliflower steaks or cook zucchini slices. The only difference will be the amount of time they cook, and they will cook evenly and at the same time if everything is cut the same.
- o Salt and pepper the vegetables before putting them into the oven and drizzle with water or vegetable stock before cooking and then check them halfway through for 20 minutes or less of cooking, or in thirds for anything that cooks for over 20 minutes, and drizzle with water once or twice and flip or stir if necessary to keep them from drying too much.
- o All vegetables are better with an acid. Either shake on lemon pepper seasoning before cooking, or squeeze lime or lemon on them just before serving. If using a fresh acid, the longer it sets on the food, the more sour it will become and, at some point, it will take on a rancid taste. Never add a fresh acid until you're ready to serve or put lime wedges on the plate. It looks nice and adds color, plus it's appealing to be able to control how much acid is in the dish to the person's personal taste.

## Cutting terms

Throughout recipes, you'll find several terms for cutting the plants to prepare them for cooking.

The most common terms used are as follows:

- Brunoise – A brunoise is the smallest dice cut and is typically first julienned and then cut into tiny cubes, usually 1 to 2 millimeters or 5/64 of an inch in size. A brunoise is used in recipes where its only purpose is to add flavor or it's used as a garnish.

- Small dice – This cut is approximately twice the size of a brunoise at a ¼ inch cube. Small dice or diced small is a term you'll find often in my recipes as it is used in several types of dishes. The onion below is an example of what I mean by dice small.

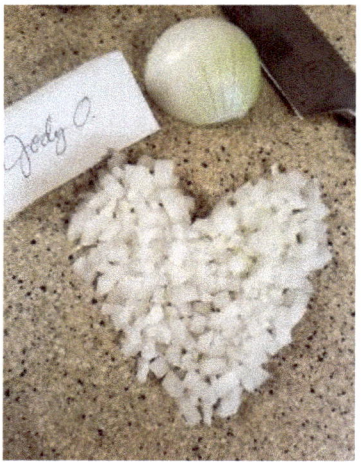

- Medium dice – This cut is ½ inch cubes and is the default size whenever a recipe says to dice an item, but doesn't specify a particular size. The following green bell pepper, celery, and tomato are examples of a medium dice.

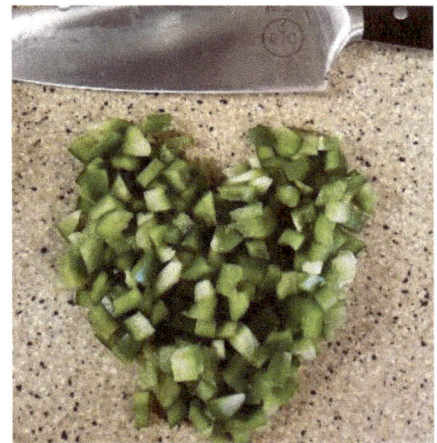

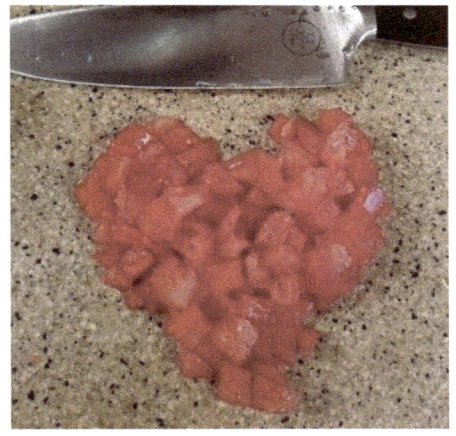

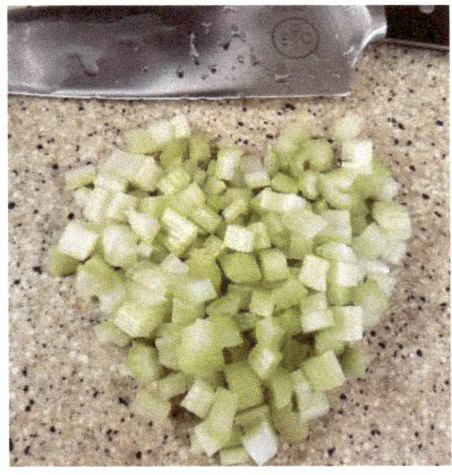

- Large dice – A large dice is typically cut into 1-inch cubes and is often used for potatoes.

- Batonnet – A batonnet cut is a stick measuring approximately ½ inch by 3 inches. The sweet potato fries in the picture below are a mixture of julienne and batonnet and some will get crispy while others stay slightly undercooked. If this is occurring while cooking fries, work on cutting the potato more evenly.

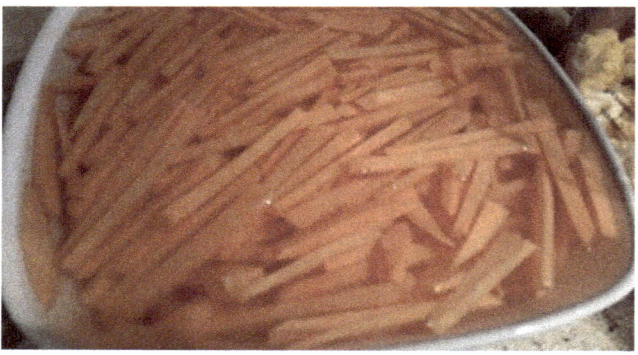

- Julienne – A julienne cut is made from a batonnet by cutting into strips lengthwise and is typically 1/8 by 3 inches. These strips are used as garnishes or in wraps.

- Fine julienne – The fine julienne cut is made from a julienne and is approximately 1/16 by 3 inches. It can be cut down for a brunoise and the strips are used for a garnish.

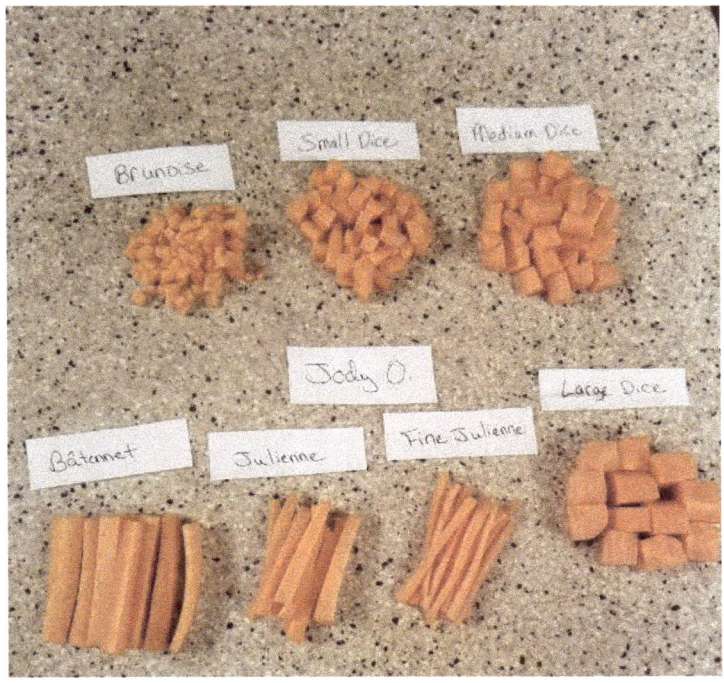

These pictures offer a visual image of the terms and display how they appear when cutting a carrot.

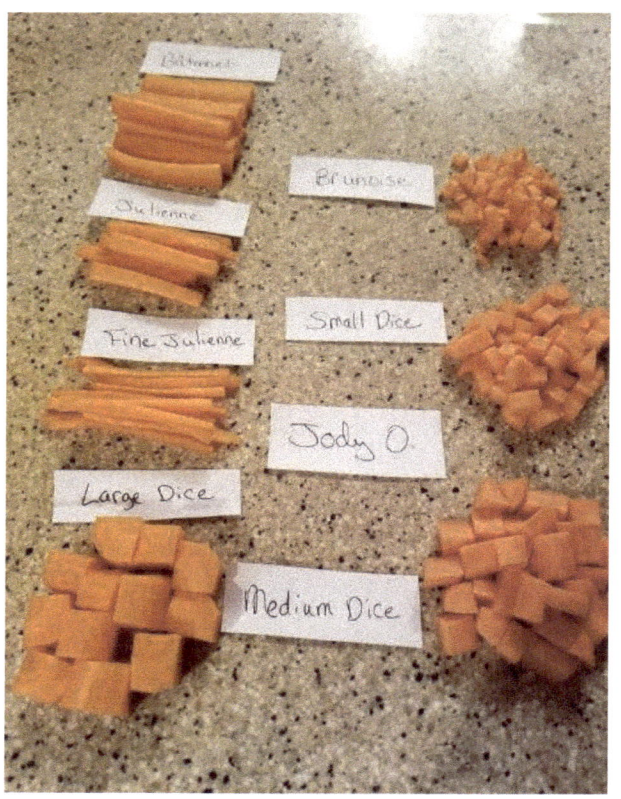

- Slice – This cucumber is sliced evenly. Notice how the bottom of the cucumber is flat. Whenever slicing something round, such as a cucumber, carrot, or potato, to make it safe to slice so that the product doesn't roll when you're cutting, causing you to accidentally cut yourself, always make one slice to cut a flat bottom, then hold it firmly in place on the flat side while slicing.

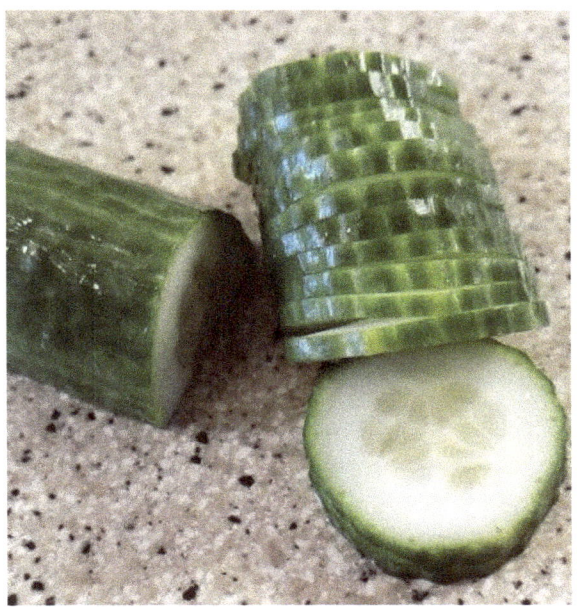

- Chop – The asparagus shows an example of what I mean by the term "chop." I cut off the tough ends and cut it into similarly sized pieces to roast evenly. I also chop herbs, which is just basically cutting them to the size I think will work best. You can use the chiffonade method, which is cutting them into long strips, but that is mostly for presentation purposes. I'm not that bougie.

- Shred - For lettuce, I shred it with my hands. Some people like to chop it. To me, it's easier and faster just to shred it into the size I like.

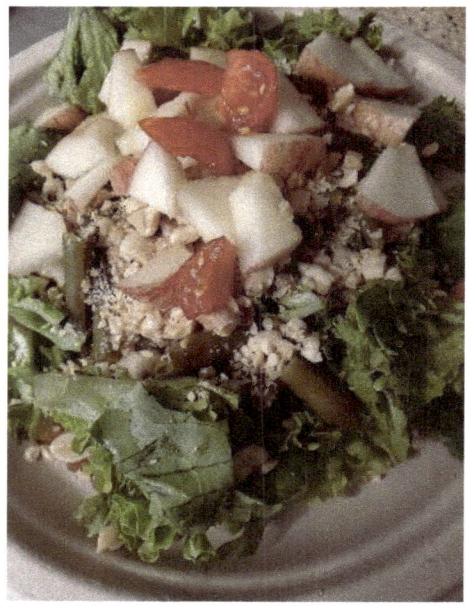

Shredded salad with chopped toppings.

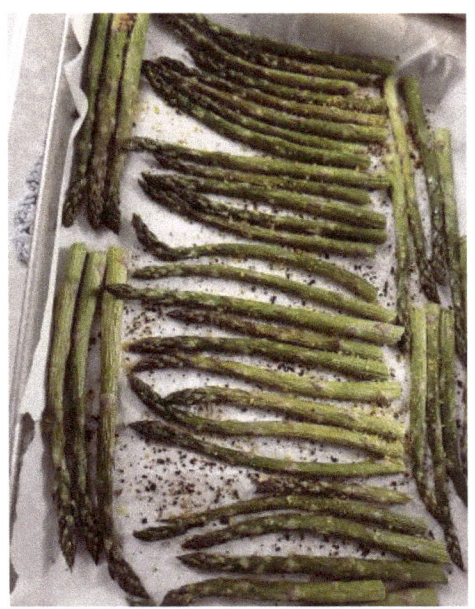

The broccoli florets are cut into similar sizes for even cooking.

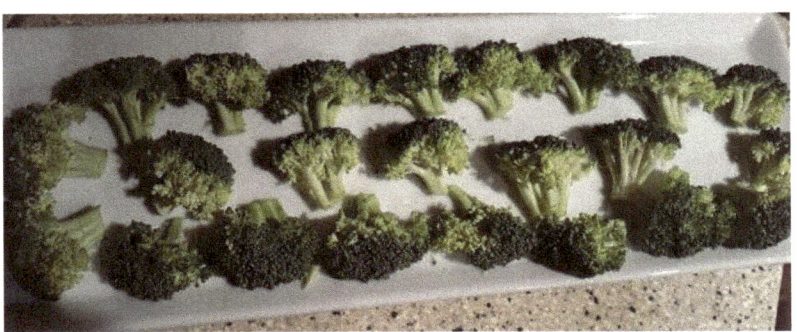

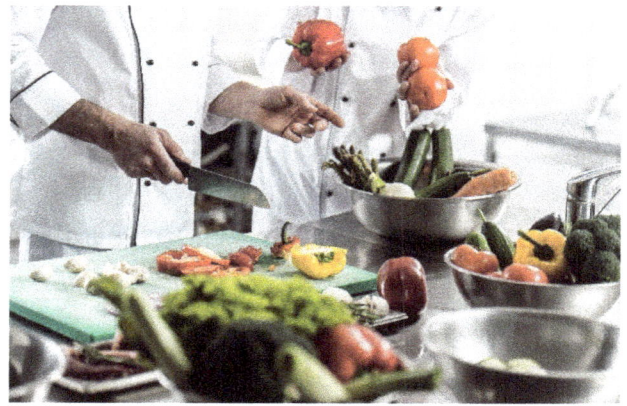

*Picture by Lightfield Studios*

# RESTAURANTS

*"People who love to eat are always the best people."*
*Julia Child*

Switching to a plant-based vegan lifestyle makes eating out challenging, unless you're fortunate enough to live in a community with enough vegans to sustain a plant-based restaurant, or at least a restaurant that is plant-based and vegan friendly.

I've found that in my city, it's necessary to educate servers, restaurant managers, and even chefs on what the term "vegan" means. I can't tell you how many times I've asked for vegan options, and the server lists off the gluten-free dishes or they say, "The pizza is vegan" and I ask for a list of ingredients, which mentions cheese. Since it has a cauliflower crust, they believe it's vegan. Restaurant staff members are accustomed to receiving requests from gluten-free patrons, but not vegans.

Be diligent! Each time I order, I go through the list of what I don't want on my food. As my husband lowers his head, I say clearly, "No oil, no dairy products including milk, cheese, and butter, no eggs, no meat whatsoever, no lard, no chicken stock, no croutons on the salad, because those usually are made with butter."

If you're not comfortable asking for changes to be made to the food and sending food back when they get it wrong, because they will, then start with vegan friendly restaurants to become practiced in looking at the menu and picking out everything that may be in the dish that you don't want to put into your body.

Also, be prepared to eat items that aren't plant-based. Some restaurants only serve vegan options like fries and that's it. My husband enjoys dining out and getting his steak fresh off the grill and multiple times I've made a plate of fries into a meal. It happens. It's not healthy, but it does happen. Just be prepared and don't beat yourself up over it, and definitely don't take your frustration out on the wait staff. Instead, use the time as an opportunity to educate the manager or owner on plant-based vegan options that they can easily incorporate into their menu so that vegans can visit their establishments with omnivorous friends and family.

**Ingredients that can sneak into your food**

- Lard – This is made from fat in the abdomen of a pig. It's a common ingredient in tortillas and refried beans at Mexican restaurants. Always ask if their beans or tortillas are made with lard. If so, skip the tortillas and ask about their black beans. Most often, black beans contain no additives.

- Chicken stock – Every Mexican restaurant in which I've dined puts chicken stock in their rice to flavor it. It's good that I have my mother-in-law's wonderful recipe for rice (included in this book), otherwise I'd crave Spanish rice because I haven't eaten it at a restaurant in years. Restaurants such as On the Border offer a cilantro lime rice that's similar to what I make on occasion at home. It's not traditional Spanish rice, but it's a good substitute. Try it.

- Egg – Restaurants love to use egg as a binding agent. They use it in pasta, bread, eggrolls (duh), and in fried rice. There are very few Italian restaurants that have vegan options in Oklahoma and if I pick up Asian food, I always make sure to tell them "no egg" in the fried rice, which is very oily so I don't eat it often. Instead of eggrolls, I order vegetable summer rolls. They're not the same texture and the sauce is a peanut sauce instead of sweet and sour, but it's a decent substitute.

- Butter – It seems that butter is in everything. It's definitely in croutons at Red Lobster. Several years ago, before I quit eating meat, my family planned to go downtown to watch the fireworks on July 4th and we ate lunch at Red Lobster, one of my husband's favorites. My daughter ordered a salad with no cheese and she told the server that she has an issue with dairy, so no dairy whatsoever on the salad. When her salad arrived, it had croutons on it. She told the server no dairy, so she trusted him and just started eating. Within 10 minutes we were running her to the bathroom where she camped out for at least a half hour before heading home and missing the fireworks. The manager felt so bad that he mailed a $75 gift card to me. At least they made up for their error. The lesson here is to never trust your server. Talk to a manager if possible if you have any issues with food, and never eat the croutons unless you're eating in a fully plant-based restaurant such as Plant in midtown Oklahoma City.

- Cheese – Again, several years ago, my family decided to go downtown and eat at a favorite spaghetti restaurant that featured train cars set up as booths so that you could dine inside the train. Their food was good, and we really enjoyed it. When ordering, my daughter asked for the spaghetti and meatballs and specified no cheese or dairy on her food. She was in luck; their spaghetti wasn't made with egg. Yay! She made it through one meatball before heading to the bathroom. We found out that the pasta sauce and meatballs contained cheese. Unlike Red Lobster, this restaurant didn't attempt to make things right. They've since gone out of business. Lesson learned? Some pasta sauces and pizza doughs contain cheese or egg. I read recently about some of the wonderful things that the owner of Little Caesars does in communities, and I wanted to support their business. I called to see if they have a vegan option and was told "no." I've had the same response from other pizza companies. No vegan options whatsoever. When we're craving pizza, we go to Whole Foods where we can eat their whole wheat crust and red sauce, plus they offer hummus as a topping, and we load them with vegetables, or we make pizza at home.

We rarely eat food from restaurants these days. Once you learn how to cook, the food often tastes better at home. But these are my top 4 choices that are available in my area and what I order.

- Plant – This restaurant offers plant-based vegan food with no soy. We can eat anything on their menu. It's the only option like it in town.

- Chick-fil-A – Since we have very few options, we stop at Chick-fil-A on occasion and order either the Market or Southwest salad bases (meaning no chicken) and with no cheese. When ordering, say "base with no cheese" and then specify "no chicken and no cheese." Their Southwest salad comes with tortilla strips that contain milk, so if possible, tell them no strips and instead request almond slivers or extra pepitas. All their salad dressings have oil or dairy or eggs. While there are a couple of vegan choices, there is no real plant-based choice. We use dressing at home or if you're okay with occasional oil, you can order the light balsamic vinaigrette. They also offer a veggie wrap, but the tortilla is white flour and I guess it depends on how strict you want to be with your diet. I ordered this option a few times with no chicken or cheese before going plant-based and I'd get home and find chicken or cheese in it. Always check your order. I check my salad every single time, because 3 out of 5 times, there will be cheese in my salad.

- Panera Bread – Their plant-based menu is deceiving. The only truly plant-based option is possibly their Ten-Vegetable soup or their side option…an apple. I order their Mediterranean Vegetable sandwich with no feta cheese and have them add spinach and cilantro and I eat the soup on the side. Since my daughter has issues with dairy and I'm allergic to it, I specify "dairy allergy" when ordering so I don't get home and find cheese in our sandwiches, but it still happens on occasion. Again, check your food.

- Outback Steakhouse – This is my husband's favorite restaurant. I order their baked potato "dry" which still comes with oil on the skin and sautéed vegetables with no butter and a side salad with only raw plant toppings.

While your options will be more limited when eating in restaurants, you'll soon discover what your local establishments have to offer vegans like you, or perhaps you can be the person who creates change for the rest of us and raise awareness to our dietary needs that are being ignored.

# ONE WEEK PLAN

*"By failing to prepare, you are preparing to fail."*
*Benjamin Franklin*

I've created for you a basic example of on one-week plan I create for my clients. When working with individuals, every plan is different as I take into consideration the amount of time you have to prepare a meal, if you need to eat it on the go, and special dietary needs and preferences.

Pay attention to portion sizes on the recipes because some will be used as leftovers for following meals.

# One-week Menu

|  | Mon | Tue | Wed | Thu | Fri | Sat | Sun |
|---|---|---|---|---|---|---|---|
| **Breakfast** | Chocolate Cashew Vegan Pudding | Chocolate Cashew Vegan Pudding (Leftover | Apple Oatmeal Bowl | Apple Oatmeal Bowl (Leftover ) | Overnight Oats | Overnight t Oats | Berry Smoothie |
| **Snack 1** | Apple Butter Almond Toast | Apple Butter Almond Toast | Apple Butter Almond Toast | Ginger bread Protein Smoothie | Spinach Dip & Zucchini Chips | Spinach Dip & Zucchini Chips (Leftover | Spinach Dip & Zucchini Chips (Leftover |
| **Lunch** | Thai Salad | Cauliflower Bowl (Leftover | Tomato Soup w/ Cabbage & Potato Bites w/ Broccoli (Leftover | Tomato Soup w/ Cabbage & Potato Bites w/ Broccoli (Leftover | Beet Burger w/ Sweet Potato Fries (Leftover | Quinoa Chili w/ Crackers (Leftover | Chick Pea Scramble (Leftover |
| **Snack 2** | Ginger Bread Protein Smoothie | Ginger Bread Protein Smoothie | Chocolate Cashew Vegan Pudding (Leftover) | Banana Nut Muffin | Banana Nut Muffin | Banana Nut Muffin | Banana Nut Muffin |
| **Dinner** | Cauli flower Bowl | Tomato Soup w/ Cabbage & Potato Bites w/ Broccoli | Thai Salad (Leftover) | Beet Burger w/ Sweet Potato Fries | Quinoa Chili w/ Crackers | Chick Pea Scramble | High Protein Cauli Flower & Broccoli Casserole |

208

## Shopping List

### Fruits

- 6 apples
- 1 avocado
- 6 bananas
- 1/3 cup strawberries
- 2 lemons
- 2 limes
- 8 medjool dates

### Baking, Nuts & Spices

- 1 ¼ cup almond butter
- 1/3 cup maple syrup
- 4 ½ cups cashews
- ½ tsp cayenne pepper
- 1/3 cup chia seeds
- 1 2/3 tbsp chili powder
- 1 ½ tbsp cinnamon
- 1 1/18 tbsp cumin
- 1 tsp dried basil
- ½ tsp garlic powder
- 1 tsp ground flax seed
- 2 tsp Italian seasoning (or a mixture of oregano, basil, & thyme)
- 1 tsp nutmeg
- ½ tsp onion powder
- 3 1/3 tbsp oregano
- ½ cup raw peanuts
- 1 ¾ tsp sea salt & black pepper
- 2 tsp smoked paprika
- 1 tsp turmeric
- ¾ cup walnuts
- 5 cups almond flour
- 1 tbsp arrowroot
- 1 tsp baking powder
- ½ cup cacao nibs
- 1 tbsp cacao powder
- ¾ cup coconut sugar
- 4 cups einkorn wheat flour
- 1/3 tsp ground cloves
- ½ cup nutritional yeast
- 2 cups oats
- 1 ½ tsp vanilla extract

### Frozen

- ½ cup frozen cauliflower

### Vegetables

- 8 cups baby or full spinach
- 2 beets (pre-cooked if possible)
- 6 cups broccoli
- 1 small to medium butternut squash
- 3 carrots
- 2 heads cauliflower
- 3 stalks celery
- ¼ cup cilantro
- 8 cloves garlic
- 1 1/8 tbsp ginger
- 2/3 cup green beans
- 3 cups green cabbage
- 2 cups mushrooms
- ½ cup red onion
- 2 cups romaine
- 2 russet potatoes
- 1 sweet potato
- 2 thai chilis

Sprouted Vegan

- ○ 4 tomatoes
- ○ 3 yellow onions
- ○ 1 yellow squash
- ○ 6 zucchinis

- ○ 10 cups water

Boxed & Canned

- ○ 1 cup black beans
- ○ 1 cup chickpeas
- ○ 2 cups lentils
- ○ 1 ½ cups mixed beans
- ○ 2 ¼ cups quinoa
- ○ ¼ cup tomato paste
- ○ 7 ½ cups vegetable broth (or follow my recipe in this book to make your own)

Bread

- ○ 9 slices whole grain bread

Cold

- ○ ¾ cup hummus
- ○ 2 ½ cup almond milk
- ○ 1 cup unsweetened coconut yogurt

Condiments

- ○ 1 ½ tsp balsamic vinegar
- ○ ¼ cup sauerkraut
- ○ 1 tbsp tahini
- ○ 1 tbsp tamari

Other

- ○ 1 cup cooked chickpeas
- ○ 2 tsp vanilla

# Chocolate Cashew Vegan Pudding

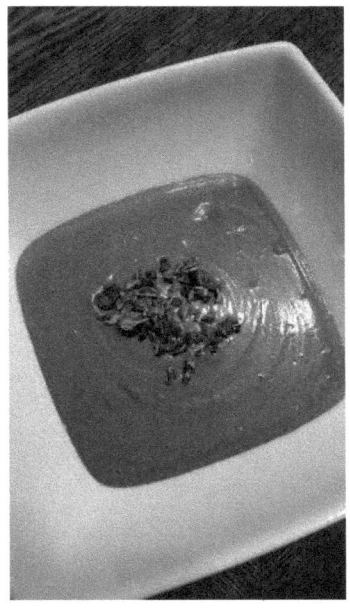

7 minutes
9 ingredients
5 servings

Ingredients

- 2 1/2 cups Almond Milk (1/2 cup extra if desired)
- 1 cup Cashews (raw)
- 1 tbsp Chia Seeds
- 1 tsp Vanilla
- 1 tbsp Arrowroot
- 1 tbsp Cacao Powder
- 1/2 cup Cacao Nibs (sweetened optional)
- 8 Medjool Dates (take out seeds)
- 1 tsp Nutmeg (freshly grated)

Instructions

1) Add all ingredients in high-speed blender.

2) Blend for 2 to 3 minutes or until smooth.

3) Add up to 1/2 cup or a little more of almond milk if it's too thick or has a grainy texture.

4) Pour into a bowl, chill, and serve with cacao nibs on top, if desired.

# Apple Oatmeal Bowl

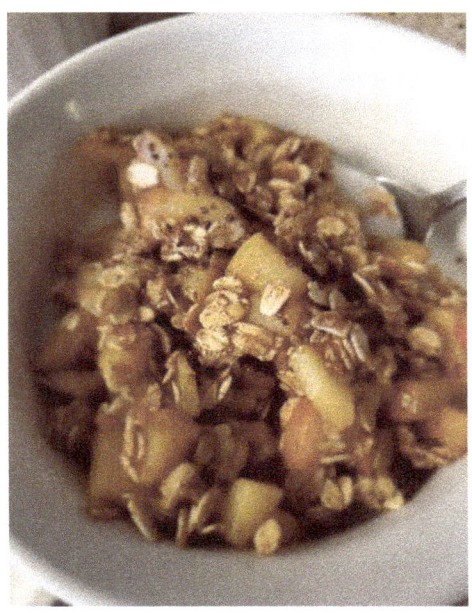

20 minutes
6 ingredients
2 servings

Ingredients
- 1 Apple (Cored and diced medium)
- 1 cup Oats
- 1 tbsp Maple Syrup
- 1 tsp Cinnamon
- 1 cup Unsweetened Coconut Yogurt
- 1/4 cup Almond Butter

Instructions
Add the apple and oats to a small pan and cook for 2 to 3 minutes, or until the apple starts to soften.
Add the maple syrup and cinnamon and continue to cook, stirring often until the oats reach desired texture, approximately 5 minutes.

Add 1/2 cup of yogurt to a bowl and top with the apple oat crisp and top with half the almond butter and serve.

# Overnight Oats

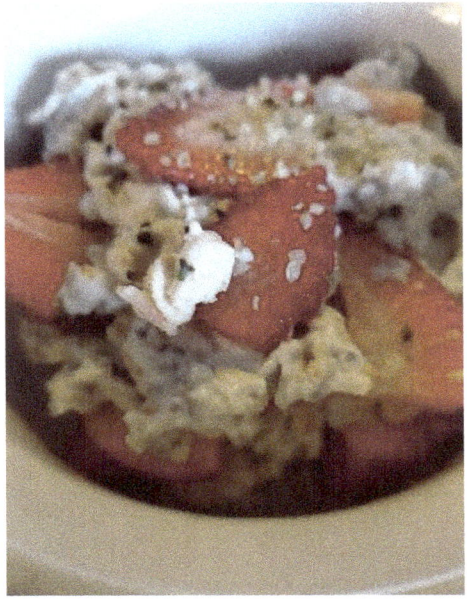

5 hours
5 ingredients
2 servings

Ingredients
- **1 cup** Oats (quick or traditional)
- **1 tbsp** Chia Seeds
- **1 1/2 cups** Oat Milk
- **1/3 cup** Strawberries
- **1 tbsp** Almond Butter

Instructions
1) In a large bowl, combine the oats, chia seeds, and milk. Stir to combine.
2) Place the mixture in the refrigerator overnight.
3) After the oats have softened, divide them into bowls to save leftovers and top with strawberries and almond butter.

# Berry Smoothie

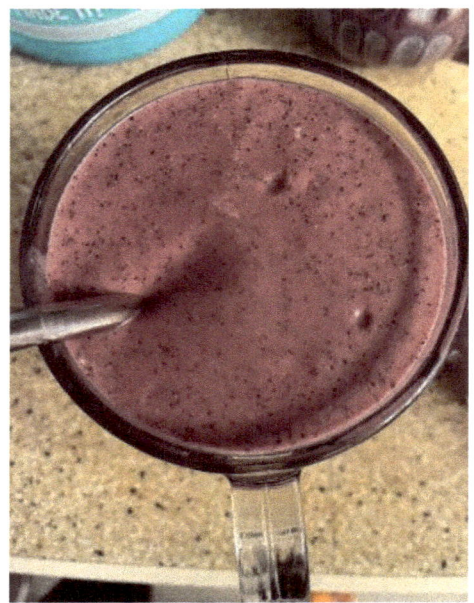

10 minutes
7 ingredients
1 serving

Ingredients
- 1/2 cup Frozen Cauliflower
- 1/2 cup Frozen Raspberries
- 1 Lemon (juiced)
- 1 tbsp Chia Seeds
- 1 cup Oat Milk
- 1 Apple (Cored and diced medium)
- 1 tsp Ginger (Fresh)

Instructions
1) Place all ingredients into your high-speed blender and blend until smooth. Add more milk if necessary to get your desired texture. Serve.

# Apple Almond Butter Toast

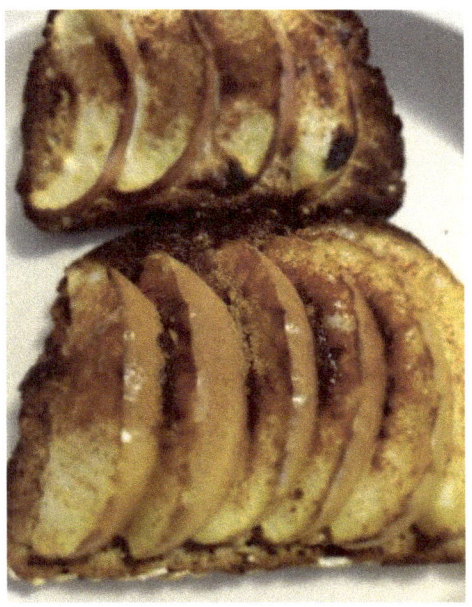

5 minutes
4 ingredients
1 serving

Ingredients
- **2 slices** Whole Grain Bread
- **1** Apple
- **1 tbsp** Almond Butter
- **1 tsp** Cinnamon

Instructions
1) Spread almond butter on bread. Place slices of bread in toaster oven.
2) Wash apple and cut into thin slices. Arrange on top of bread slices and top with cinnamon.
3) Air fry at 400 for approximately 4 minutes or until desired color. Serve.

# Gingerbread Protein Smoothie

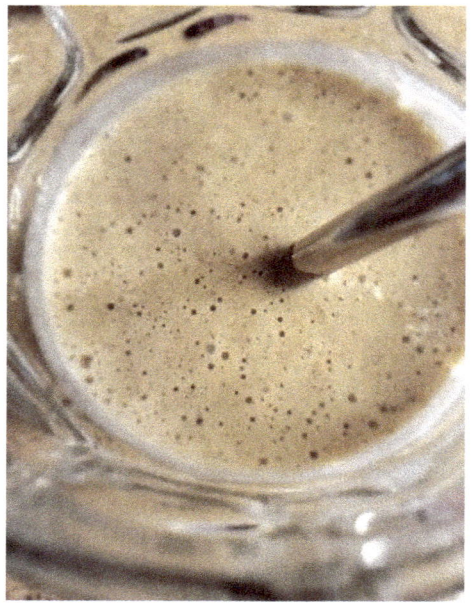

5 minutes
9 ingredients
1 serving

Ingredients

- 1 cup Oat Milk
- ½ Banana (frozen)
- 1 tbsp Chia Seeds
- 3 tbsps Almond Butter
- 1/2 tsp Vanilla Extract
- 1 1/2 tbsps Maple Syrup
- 1/2 tsp Ginger (fresh, minced)
- 1/4 tsp Cinnamon (ground)
- 1/8 tsp Ground Cloves

Instructions

1) Add everything to a high-speed blender for approximately 1 minute or until blended thoroughly. Serve.

218

# Spinach Dip & Zucchini Chips

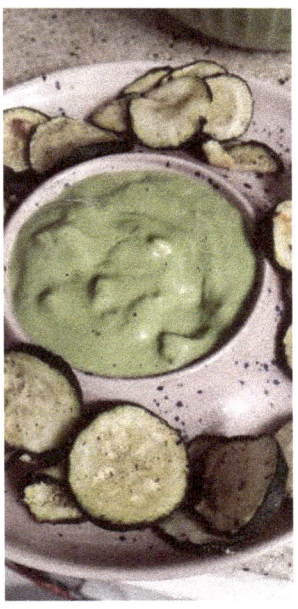

15 minutes
7 ingredients
4 servings

Ingredients
- 2 Zucchini (Sliced thin)
- 1 Sea Salt & Black Pepper (To taste)
- 1 cup Cashews
- 2 cups Baby Spinach
- 1/4 cup Lime Juice (The juice of one lime)
- 1 tbsp Oregano
- 1/2 cup Water

Instructions
1) Preheat oven to 400 or prepare air fryer. I prefer to use the air fryer. If using your oven, line a baking sheet with parchment paper.
2) Wash and slice zucchini thinly and place on baking sheet or in air fryer. Top with salt, pepper, and oregano and bake for approximately 15 minutes and

219

air fry for approximately 5 minutes or until desired texture. You want the slices crispy to be able to hold dip.

3) Add cashews, lime juice, spinach, water, and salt and pepper to a high-speed blender. Blend and add more water or cashews until you reach the desired consistency.

4) Serve on chip and dip plate or however you like to eat your chips and dips. I like my dip in a bowl of some type. Enjoy!

5) Store leftovers in airtight container in the refrigerator. Either bake or put your chips in an air fryer for just a few minutes when eating this snack to restore their crispiness.

# Thai Salad

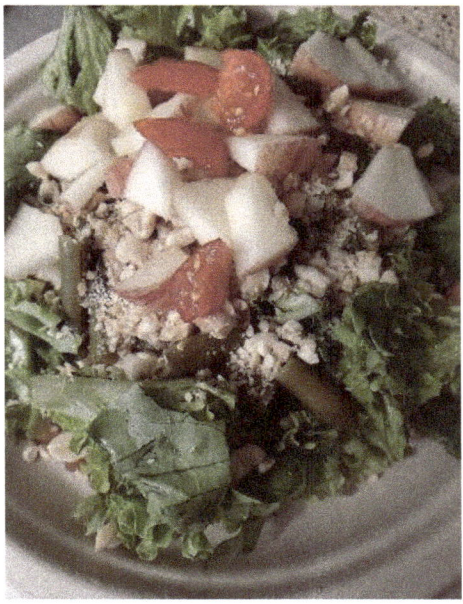

15 minutes – 25 if you don't have pre-cooked quinoa
11 ingredients
2 servings

## Ingredients

- **2 cups** Quinoa (Pre-cooked)
- **2/3 cup** Green Beans (Stemmed and chopped medium)
- **2 cups** Romaine (Washed, dried, and torn into bite-sized pieces. If you have CAD, sauté kale in a pan for 3 minutes stirring constantly with no oil and use instead.)
- **2** Thai Chili (Stemmed and diced small)
- **1** Tomato (Diced small)
- **1/2 cup** Raw Peanuts (Chopped small or whole)
- **1 tbsp** Maple Syrup
- **1 tbsp** Tamari
- **2** Garlic (Minced cloves)
- **½** Lime (juiced)

221

- 1 Apple (Cored and diced medium)

Instructions
1) Cook the quinoa according to package directions if you don't already have quinoa cooked.
2) Portion out half the quinoa on a plate. Save the other half for leftovers. Top with romaine or kale.
3) Top the quinoa with all the ingredients.
4) Serve.

# Cauliflower Bowl

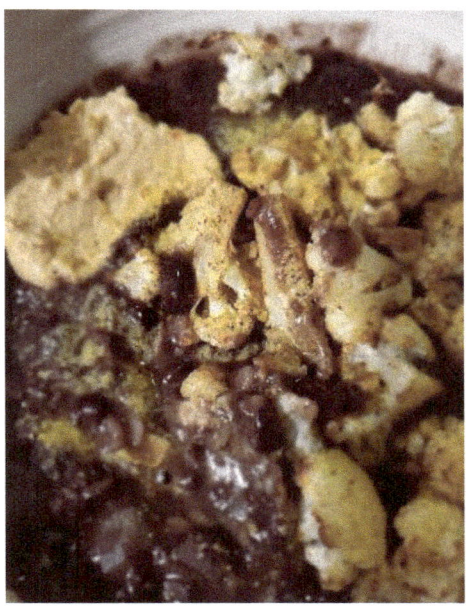

35 minutes
11 ingredients
2 servings

Ingredients

- **1 head** Cauliflower (Small head cut into florets)
- **1 1/2 tsps** Cumin
- **1/2 tsp** Chili Powder
- **1 1/2 tsps** Smoked Paprika
- **1 tsp** Sea Salt
- **1/2 cup** Water
- **1 cup** Black Beans (Cooked or canned)
- **1** Garlic (1 clove, minced)
- **1/4 cup** Cilantro
- **1 tsp** Lime Juice
- **1** Avocado

Instructions

1) Preheat your oven to 425 and line a baking sheet with parchment paper. Toss the cauliflower with the cumin, half the chili powder, half the smoked paprika and half the sea salt.

2) Place the cauliflower inside the oven and cook for approximately 20 minutes or until tender. Turn it over halfway.

3) Mash the beans with a pastry cutter or fork. Add the beans to a small pan along with the water and the remaining spices and cook on low heat for approximately 5 minutes.

4) In a small bowl, add the avocado and lime juice and mash the mixture. Add salt and pepper to taste.

5) Remove the cauliflower from the oven and divide your portion for this meal and your leftovers for lunch. Add half the beans and top with your homemade guacamole and cilantro. If you have sour cream made (in the recipe section), also top with a spoonful of sour cream. Store your leftovers in airtight containers in the refrigerator.

# Tomato Soup with Cabbage

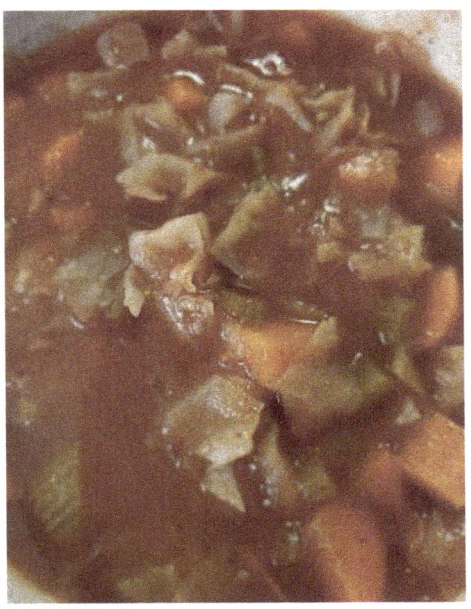

45 minutes
12 ingredients
4 servings

Ingredients

- 1/4 cup Water
- 1 Yellow Onion (small)
- 3 stalks Celery (Diced small)
- 3 Carrot (Peeled and diced small)
- 1 Garlic (2 medium or 1 large clove, minced)
- 1 Sea Salt & Black Pepper (To taste)
- 2 tsps Italian Seasoning
- 1 ½ Tomato (Cut out seeds and blend most of it, saving about 1/4 cup to add to soup diced small.)
- 3 cups Green Cabbage (Chopped)
- 6 cups Vegetable Broth
- 3 tbsps Tomato Paste (Or 1 small can)
- 1 cup Chickpeas

Instructions

1) In a large pot over high heat, add the onion, celery, carrot, and garlic and cook for about five minutes until the onions begin to soften. Add the water by the tablespoon to deglaze the pan if the onion sticks. Stir in the seasonings and cook until the onion turns translucent, about 3 minutes.

2) Add the rest of the ingredients and turn the heat down to medium.

3) Simmer the soup for approximately 20 minutes or until the cabbage has reached your desired tenderness. Serve.

# Potato Bites with Broccoli

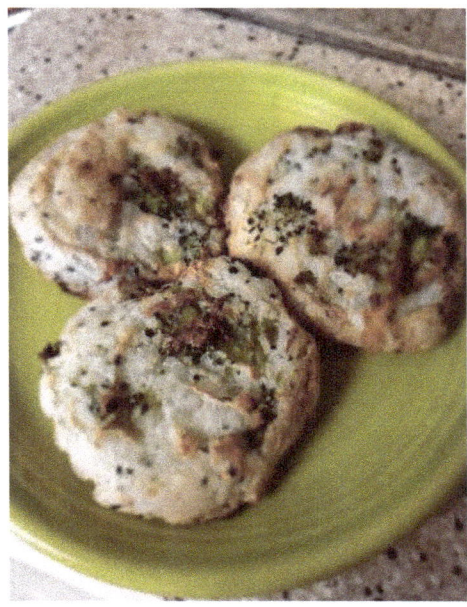

1 hour
7 ingredients
4 servings

Ingredients
- **2** Russet Potato (Peeled and diced medium)
- **2 cups** Broccoli (Cut into 1 inch pieces)
- **1/2 tsp** Onion Powder
- **1/2 tsp** Garlic Powder
- **1/4 tsp** Sea Salt
- **4 cups** Water (Enough to cover potatoes to boil and then to boil broccoli.)
- **1/2 cup** Hummus

Instructions
1) Boil the potatoes in a small pot until fork tender.
2) Add the broccoli to the potatoes and boil for approximately 3 minutes or until it's tender and the potatoes are tender enough to mash with a fork.

227

Drain all the water and remove from the heat and set aside to cool.

3) Preheat the oven to 425 and line a baking sheet with parchment paper or prepare an air fryer at 400. I tried cooking these in the oven and in the air fryer and the air fryer was 3 times faster.

4) Pour the potato mixture into a bowl and mash with a fork.

5) Add the seasoning and then form the mixture into small bite-sized patties and place on the parchment paper and in the oven for approximately 30 minutes or in the air fryer for approximately 10 minutes. Turn them over when halfway through. Serve on the side of a meal or with your favorite vegan oil-free sauce or hummus.

# Beet Burger

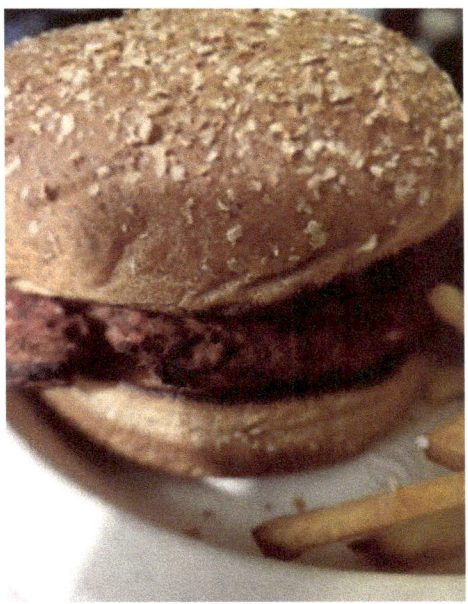

45 minutes
12 ingredients
2 servings

## Ingredients

- **2** Beet (Diced into small cubes or pre-cooked beets)
- **1 1/2 tsps** Balsamic Vinegar
- **1 tbsp** Arrowroot Powder
- **1 1/2 cups** Lentils (Cooked or canned and drained)
- **1/4 cup** Walnuts (Chopped small)
- **1 tsp** Ground Flax Seed
- **1** Garlic (1 minced clove)
- **1 tbsp** Tahini
- **1** Sea Salt & Black Pepper (To taste)
- **1/4 cup** Sauerkraut
- **1 tbsp** Water
- **1/4 cup** Hummus (Optional topping)

Instructions

1) Boil beets in small saucepan until tender if you didn't buy the pre-cooked.
2) In a small bowl, add the water, tahini, and balsamic vinegar and stir to mix. Place the bowl in the refrigerator until you're ready to use it.
3) Preheat the oven to 425 and line a baking sheet with parchment paper or prepare your air fryer at 400.
4) Add all remaining ingredients (except the sauerkraut) and cooked beets into a food processor and pulse until just crumbly. Add water as necessary to make the burgers hold their shape.
5) Form the mixture into 2 bun-sized patties or 3 if you have enough and bake for 30 minutes or air fry for 10 minutes, flipping halfway.
6) Serve these on a kale salad or on a whole grain bun and top with sauerkraut and your favorite toppings.

# Sweet Potato Fries

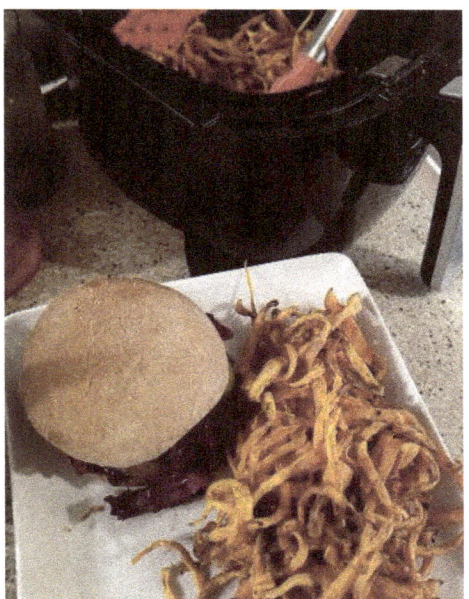

25 minutes
3 ingredients
2 servings

Ingredients
- 1 Sweet Potato (1 large sweet potato peeled and cut into battonet strips (see chef secrets chapter))
- 1 Sea Salt & Black Pepper (To taste)
- 1 tbsp Water

Instructions
1) Preheat oven to 400 degrees or prepare your air fryer. If baking, line a baking sheet with parchment paper.
2) Peel and wash your sweet potato and cut it into batonnet strips (or french fry size).
3) Place the strips onto the baking sheet or in the air fryer and top with salt, pepper, and a drizzle of water and bake or fry. Turning halfway in oven and every 5

minutes in air fryer to keep them from burning. Cook until tender, approximately 15 minutes in the oven and 10 in the air fryer. Serve.

# Quinoa Chili

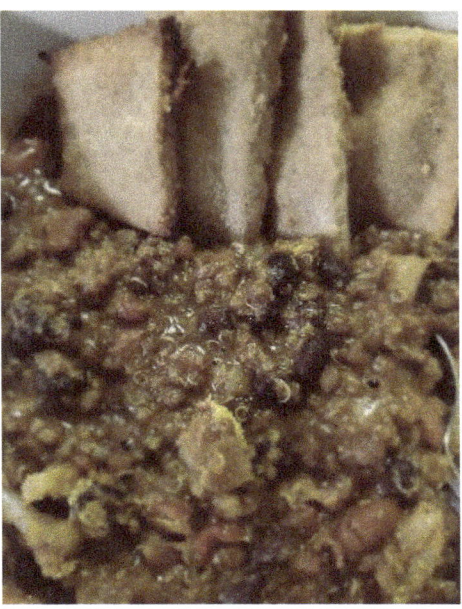

30 minutes
10 ingredients
2 servings

## Ingredients

- 1 1/2 cups Mixed Beans
- 1 Tomato (Remove seeds and dice medium)
- 1 cup Vegetable Broth (Or water)
- 1/2 cup Red Onion (Diced small)
- 1/4 cup Quinoa
- 1 Garlic (Minced)
- 1 tbsp Tomato Paste
- 1 1/2 tbsps Chili Powder
- 2 tsps Cumin
- 1 Sea Salt & Black Pepper (To taste)

## Instructions

1) Add all ingredients to a small pot and cook on medium heat for approximately 20 minutes or until

the quinoa is tender. Add more water or stock if necessary.

2) Serve.

# Crackers

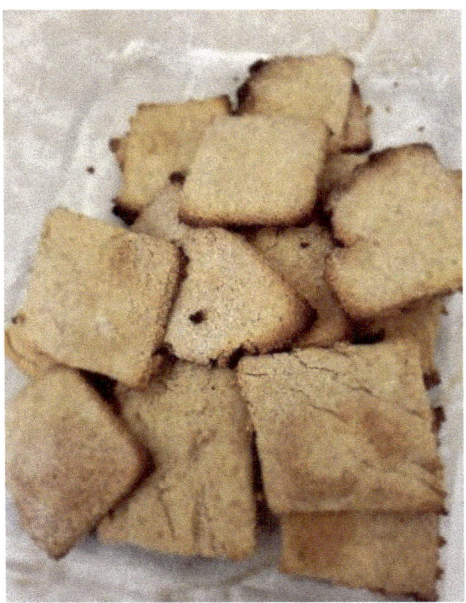

20 minutes
6 ingredients
4 servings

Ingredients
- 2 cups Almond Flour
- 1 cup Einkorn Wheat Flour
- 1 tsp Arrowroot Powder
- 1/2 tsp Oregano
- 1/2 tsp Dried Basil
- 1 cup Water

Instructions
1) Preheat the oven to 450. Mix all the ingredients in a large mixing bowl. Add more water by the teaspoon if necessary to achieve a doughy texture that holds together and doesn't flake, but isn't too sticky.
2) Sprinkle flour onto a flat surface to roll out the dough.

3) Break the dough into 2 pieces and roll it out until it's a thin square. If you want perfectly square crackers, trim the sides. If you like the artisan look, leave the sides ragged and cut into approximately 3-inch squares and put on a parchment lined baking sheet or in an air fryer if you have one with a large flat basket.

4) Bake in oven for approximately 7 minutes, turning halfway, or in an air fryer for approximately 5 minutes or until desired crispness.

5) Serving size is approximately 4 crackers.

# Chickpea Scramble

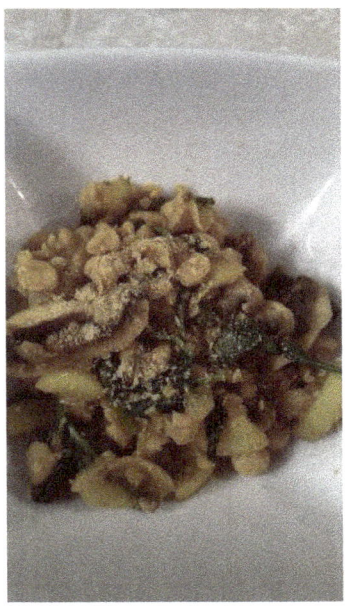

15 minutes
13 ingredients
2 servings

Ingredients

- **1 cup** Cooked Chickpeas (Mash the chickpeas before adding them to the pan if you want a scrambled egg consistency.)
- **¼** Yellow Onion (Diced)
- **1** Yellow Squash (peeled and sliced)
- **1 clove** Garlic (minced)
- **2 cups** Mushrooms (Washed and sliced)
- **½** Lemon (juiced)
- **2 cups** Spinach
- **1 tsp** Turmeric
- **1 tsp** Ginger (Grated)
- **1 tbsp** Nutritional Yeast
- **1/2 cup** Vegetable Broth
- **1/2 tsp** Cayenne Pepper
- Sea Salt & Black Pepper (to taste)

237

Instructions
1) Heat pan over high heat.
2) Add diced onions and stir continuously until translucent.
3) Add garlic and mushrooms and continue to stir until it starts to stick to the pan.
4) Add just enough vegetable broth to keep it from sticking.
5) Toss in chickpeas, squash, turmeric, salt, pepper, and cayenne, if using.
6) Continue to stir for about 1 minute.
7) Grate ginger over top and pour in the remaining vegetable broth.
8) Toss in spinach and cook until it starts to wilt, stirring occasionally.
9) Stir and serve with sprinkled nutritional yeast and lemon juice squeezed on top.

# Banana Nut Muffins

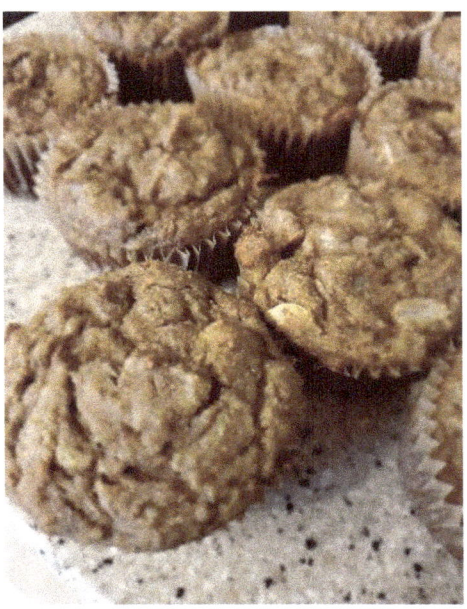

25 minutes
10 ingredients
12 servings

Ingredients

- **1 cup** Almond Flour
- **2 cups** Einkorn Wheat Flour
- **1/2 tsp** Sea Salt
- **1 tsp** Baking Powder
- **1 tsp** Vanilla
- **3/4 cup** Coconut Sugar
- **1/2 cup** Walnuts
- **4** Bananas (Over ripe)
- **1/4 cup** Arrowroot Powder (Or Tapioca flour)
- **1 cup** Water

Instructions
1) Preheat oven to 350 degrees.

2) Line cupcake pan with 12 parchment paper cupcake cups.

3) In a large mixing bowl, mash bananas then add all the dry ingredients. Mix by hand.

4) Add all the other ingredients to the mixture, adding more water by the tablespoon until you get a thick, wet consistency. You should be able to easily stir the mixture, but it shouldn't be like liquid.

5) Pour the mixture into the cups using a 1/4 cup measuring cup.

6) Bake muffins at 350 for approximately 12 to 15 minutes or until they feel firm and are a light golden color on top. Remove from the oven and allow to cool outside of the pan for at least 5 minutes before serving. The longer they cool, the less they will stick to the paper.

# High Protein Cauliflower & Broccoli Casserole

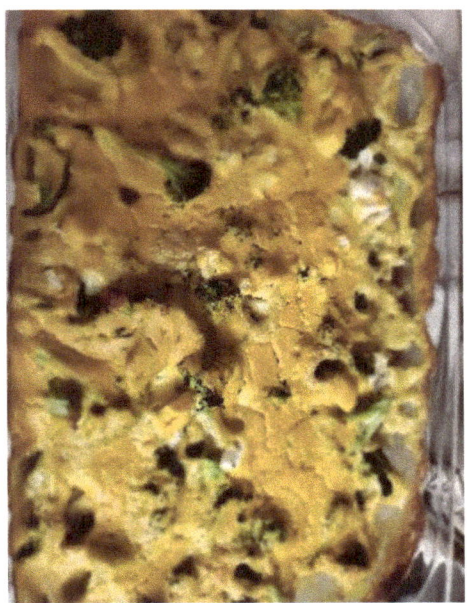

50 minutes
11 ingredients
4 servings

Ingredients

- **3 cups** Butternut Squash (1 whole squash peeled, seeds removed, and diced medium)
- **1** Yellow Onion (Diced small)
- **2** Garlic (Minced)
- **1/2 cup** Water
- **1 head** Cauliflower (Cut into florets)
- **4 cups** Broccoli (Cut into florets)
- **1/2 cup** Cashews
- **1** Sea Salt & Black Pepper (To taste)
- **1/2 tsp** Smoked Paprika
- **1/2 cup** Nutritional Yeast
- **1/2 cup** Lentils

Instructions
1) Preheat oven to 375.
2) Bring a large pan to high heat and add the onions. Cook for approximately 1 minute, stirring constantly, then add the garlic and cook for an additional 3 minutes or until the onion is translucent. Stir constantly and add 1 tablespoon of water if it sticks to the pan. Stir in the squash, lentils, and water and cook until the lentils are tender.
3) Fill a medium-sized pot halfway with water and bring water to a boil. Add the squash and cauliflower and boil for approximately 4 minutes or until just tender. Drain immediately.
4) Add the lentils and squash to a high-speed blender and blend until just mixed. If you don't have a Vitamix, add more water or use a food processor.
5) Using a rectangle baking dish, spread the broccoli and cauliflower on the bottom and then cover with the sauce from the lentils and squash.
6) Bake for 40 minutes. Serve.

# Bonus Holiday Recipes

These are a few of my favorite holiday recipes and they are a tradition in my home. The items on the list are staples that I keep on hand. Once you stock your kitchen with plant-based basics, you won't need to purchase as many items. This menu feeds 8.

These recipes are plant-based versions of the classics, and every new client receives something that looks similar to this format, along with a shopping list, every week when they receive their plans. Enjoy!

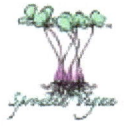

## Holiday Menu

Created by Sprouted Vegan

**Holiday menu
shopping list**

Fruits

- o 1 apple
- o 5 medjool dates
- o 1 1/3 tbsp orange zest

Vegetables

- o 1 medium butternut squash
- o 10 stalks celery
- o 2 tbsp fresh sage
- o 3 cloves garlic
- o 14 oz green beans
- o 2 green chili peppers (or a small can of Hatch chilis)
- o 3 russet potatoes
- o 4 sweet potatoes
- o 2 tbsp thyme
- o 3 yellow onion

Baking

- o ¼ cup maple syrup
- o 3 ½ cups almond flour
- o 1 tsp baking soda
- o 1/3 cup brown sugar (vegan brand)
- o ½ cup coconut sugar
- o ¼ tsp ground cloves
- o 2 tbsp nutritional yeast
- o 1/3 cup tapioca flour
- o 1 tsp vanilla extract

Boxed & Canned

- o 1 lb cooked chickpeas (or two cans)
- o 1 can ginger ale

- o   1 ½ cups vegetable broth

## Seeds, Nuts, & Spices
- o   1 tbsp chia seeds
- o   2 ½ tsp cinnamon
- o   1 tsp cumin
- o   1 tsp dried thyme
- o   1 tsp garlic powder
- o   1 tsp ground allspice
- o   ½ tsp ground mustard
- o   1 1/3 tsp ground sage
- o   1 tsp nutmeg
- o   ¾ cup pecans
- o   ¾ tsp sea salt & black pepper
- o   1 cup slivered almonds
- o   1 tsp smoked paprika

## Bread

- o   20 slices whole grain bread

## Cold
- o   2 ½ cups almond milk
- o   2 ¼ cups orange juice

## Other
- o   1 cup dried fig
- o   5 cups water

# Sweet Potato Casserole

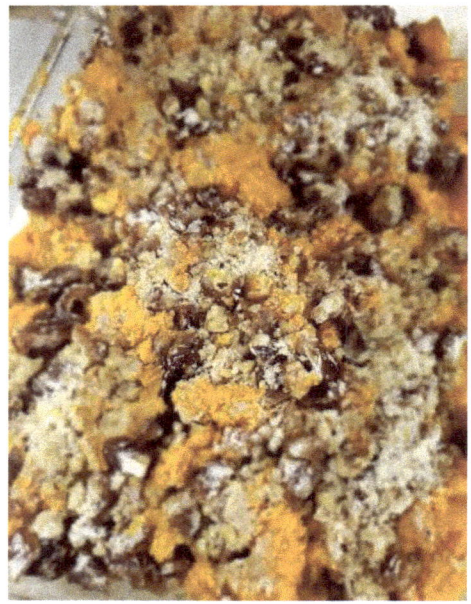

9 ingredients · 35 minutes · 8 servings

Ingredients

- 4 Sweet Potato (Washed and peeled)
- 1/2 cup Coconut Sugar
- 3 tbsps Brown Sugar
- 2 tbsps Tapioca Flour (Or arrowroot)
- tsp Vanilla Extract
- 1/2 tsp Cinnamon
- cups Almond Milk
- 3/4 cup Pecans (Chopped)
- 1/2 cup Almond Flour

Directions

1) Add sweet potatoes to large pot of boiling water. Boil until tender. Remove, drain, and cool.
2) Preheat oven to 400.
3) Line a rectangular or large baking pan with parchment paper to keep the food from sticking to the pan.
4) Mash the sweet potatoes with a fork and add to large mixing bowl. Add all remaining ingredients except the chopped pecans and mix with a stand mixer or by hand until thoroughly mixed.
5) Fold in chopped pecans with a spoon.
6) Pour the mixture into baking pan and bake for approximately 20 minutes or until golden on top. Let cool and serve.

# Dressing

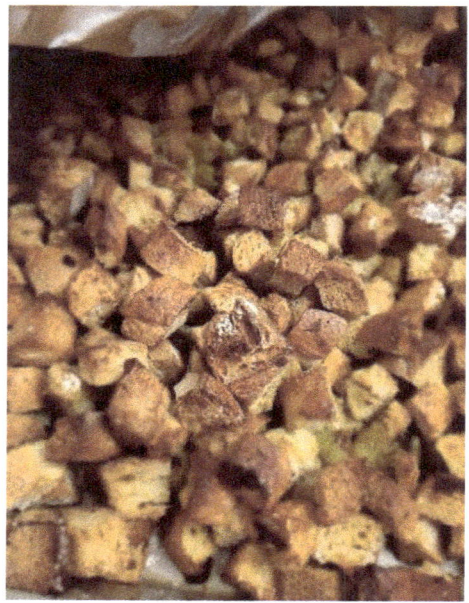

9 ingredients · 45 minutes · 10 servings

Ingredients

- 20 slices Whole Grain Bread (Cut into cubes)
- 2 Yellow Onion (Diced)
- 10 stalks Celery (sliced)
- 2 tbsps Fresh Sage (chopped)
- 2 tbsps Thyme (chopped)
- 1 tsp Nutmeg (fresh ground)
- 1 tbsp Ground Sage
- 1 tsp Sea Salt & Black Pepper
- 4 cups Water

Directions

1) Preheat the oven to 400 degrees.
2) In a medium sized saucepan, add water, onion, celery, and ground sage, bring to a boil and turn down the heat to a simmer until onions are tender. Add more water as necessary,
3) Add breadcrumbs and all the ingredients to a large roasting pan with salt and pepper. Mix well, ensuring that all bread crumbs are moist. Add more water if necessary but not to the point of standing liquid in the pan.
4) Bake the dressing for approximately 30 to 45 minutes or until cooked to desired texture. Let cool and serve.

# Cranberry Sauce

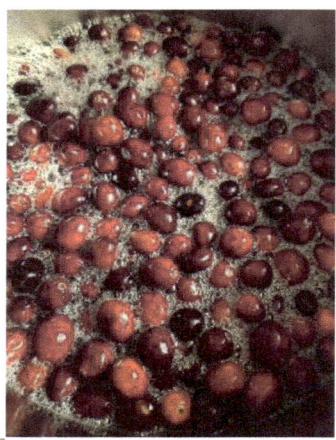

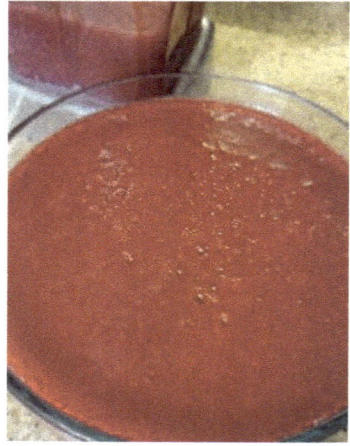

7 ingredients · 40 minutes · 10 servings

Ingredients

- 1 ½ cups Frozen Cranberries (Can use fresh cranberries, which I prefer)
- 2 cups Orange Juice
- 1 can Ginger Ale
- 2 Tbsp Maple Syrup
- 2 Tbsp Brown Sugar

- 1 Tbsp Orange Zest
- ½ tsp Sea Salt

Directions

1) Add all ingredients to large pot.
2) Bring to boil.
3) Reduce heat to medium and simmer for 30 minutes.
4) Skim stuff off the top.
5) Pour into blender and blend.
6) Serve.

# Spicy Green Beans

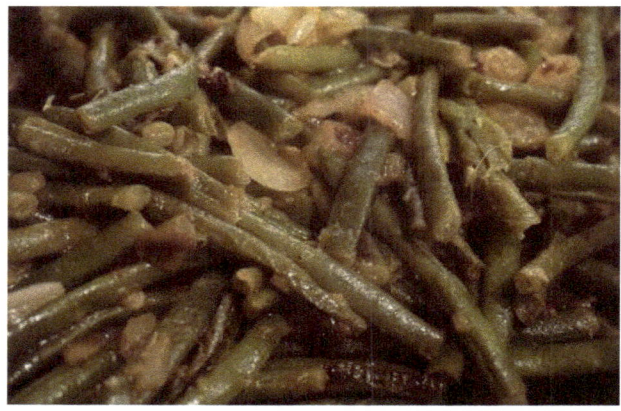

7 ingredients · 15 minutes · 6 servings

## Ingredients

- **14 ozs** Green Beans (Approximately 4 cups of green beans)
- **1/2 tsp** Ground Mustard
- **3 cloves** Garlic (Minced)
- 1 Yellow Onion (Diced fine)
- **1 tsp** Cumin (Ground cumin)
- **1/4 tsp** Sea Salt
- 2 Green Chili Pepper (Diced fine, can also use a small can of Hatch green chilies)

## Directions

1) Wash and trim green bean stems.
2) Heat large skillet to high heat.
3) Add garlic, green chilies, onion, salt, and mustard seed and stir constantly for about 1 minute or until the onion is translucent.

252

4) Add green beans. Continue to stir constantly until the beans are cooked to desired consistency. I like my beans crisp, but my husband prefers limp green beans, as seen in the picture. Cooking time is just a point of preference. Serve.

# Holiday Chickpea Patties

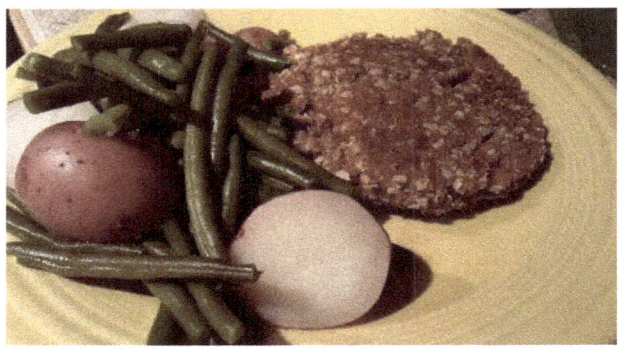

11 ingredients · 45 minutes · 8 servings

## Ingredients

- 1 lb Cooked Chickpeas (Approximately 1 can or
- 16 oz of freshly cooked)
- cups Butternut Squash (Peeled and cut into small cubes)
- cup Almond Flour
- tbsp Tapioca Flour
- 1 tsp Garlic Powder
- 1 tsp Smoked Paprika
- 1 tsp Ground Sage
- 1 tsp Dried Thyme
- 1/2 tsp Sea Salt & Black Pepper
- 2 tbsps Nutritional Yeast
- 1/2 cup Vegetable Broth (Can substitute water)

## Directions

1) Heat oven to 425.

254

2) Peel butternut squash and dice into small cubes.
3) Spread squash onto baking sheet with parchment paper and coat with salt, pepper, and 2 tablespoons of vegetable stock.
4) Cook squash for approximately 25 to 30 minutes in 425 f degree oven or until tender. Remove from oven and cool for approx 5 minutes.
5) Put everything except almond flour and vegetable stock into food processor until blended. If you like chunky patties, I use a potato masher or dough cutter in a bowl and blend and mash by hand.
6) Add flour and 1 tablespoon at a time of stock or water if necessary to make patties stick together.
7) Put nonstick frying pan on stove over high heat.
8) With your hands, create a ball with the mixture, then flatten into patty. Continue, makes about 8 patties.
9) Heat frying pan until pan is very hot. A sprinkle of water should turn into a mercury ball.
10) Fry patties for about 3 to 4 minutes on each side until brown. If the patties start to burn, turn the heat down to medium once you've browned both sides.
11) Top with A1 or your favorite sauce or gravy.

# Mashed Potatoes

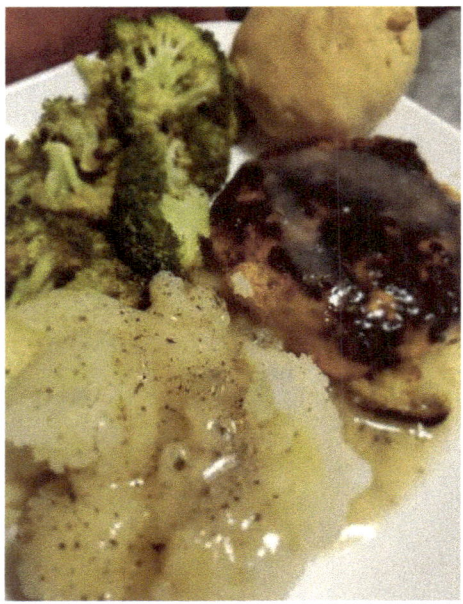

3 ingredients · 25 minutes · 8 servings

Ingredients

- 3 lbs Russet Potato (Approximately 6 large potatoes)
- 1 cup Vegetable Broth
- 1 tsp Sea Salt & Black Pepper

Directions

1) Bring a large pot of water to a boil.
2) Wash and peel potatoes. Cut into large cubes and put into a large bowl of cold water while cutting and until the water in the pan is boiling. This will help to

remove extra starch. (The more evenly the potatoes cubes are cut, the more evenly they'll cook and be tender at the same time.)

3) Drain and rinse the potato cubes and add them to the pot of water and boil until tender. Approximately 20 minutes.

4) Drain the water from the potatoes and put into a stand mixing bowl or leave in the pot if mixing by hand.

5) Add vegetable stock, salt, and pepper. Mix until desired creaminess. Add water if necessary to make them creamier. Serve.

# Figgy Pudding

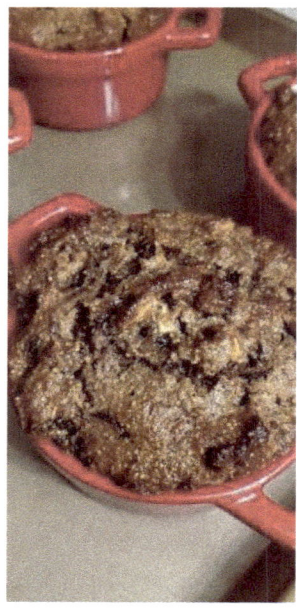

17 ingredients · 40 minutes · 5 servings

Ingredients

- 1 cup Dried Fig (Chopped)
- 1/2 cup Water (Or Brandy. I prefer Brandy!~)
- 1 cup Slivered Almonds
- 2 cups Almond Flour
- 1/2 cup Frozen Cranberries (Or fresh)
- 1 cup Apple (Peeled and chopped into small cubes)
- 1/2 cup Unsweetened Almond Milk
- 1/4 cup Orange Juice
- 1 Tbsp Chia Seeds (Ground)
- 2 Tbsp Tapioca Flour (or Arrowroot)
- 2 Tbsp Maple Syrup

- 1 tsp Orange Zest
- 2 tsp Cinnamon
- 1 tsp Ground Allspice
- 1 tsp Baking Soda
- 1/4 tsp Ground Cloves
- 5 Medjool Dates

Directions
1) Preheat oven to 350.
2) Line ramekins or small baking or Bundt pan with parchment paper.
3) In a food processor, add figs, brandy (or water), almonds, almond flour, cranberries, and apples. Pulse until just combined and still slightly chunky.
4) Put the mixture into a mixing bowl and add the remaining ingredients. Mix by hand with a large spoon.
5) Put into ramekins or pan and bake for 20 approximately 20 minutes for ramekins or 35 for a larger pan or until spongy and golden brown on top.
6) Remove from the oven and let sit on cooling rack for approximately 5 minutes before serving.

# RECIPES

More recipes…I cook with my heart, not a measuring cup or spoon. So, please adjust as necessary for your taste.

## Breakfast

# Banana Nut Muffins

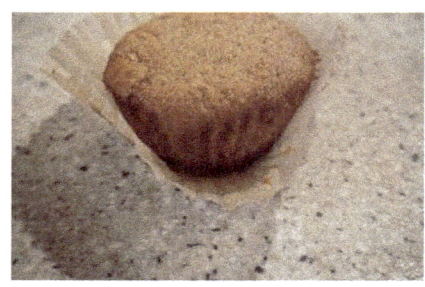

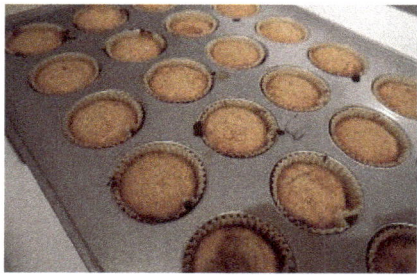

Yield 12 muffins
Time: 25 minutes

Ingredients
- 3 cups flour - I use 2 cups of home milled einkorn wheat mixed with almond flour. For gluten free, you can use brown rice flour mixed with almond.
- Pinch of kosher salt
- 1 teaspoon baking powder
- ½ teaspoon vanilla

- ¼ cup vegan sugar - not all sugar is vegan. Surprise! Make sure it's a vegan sugar. I use raw sugar.
- ½ cup crushed walnuts
- 4 overripe bananas
- 1 cup water mixed with 2 tablespoons egg replacer or arrowroot or tapioca flour– add more water as needed to get desired consistency. It should be thick and not watery.

Optional:
- ¼ cup cacao nibs
- 4 medjool dates, chopped into small pieces
- ¼ cup flax seed, optional

## Instructions
1) Preheat oven to 350 degrees
2) Line muffin pan with parchment paper baking cups. These are nonstick so you can make muffins without oil and they won't stick.
3) Sift baking soda and salt into flour in a medium sized mixing bowl
4) Mix egg replacer with water, sugar, and vanilla
5) Add egg replacer to sugar
6) Mix in mashed bananas
7) Fold in flour
8) Fold in nuts, cocoa nibs, and flax if using
9) If mixture is too runny, add more flour. If too dry, add water. Mixture should be thick and pour easily, but not runny.
10) Fill baking cups halfway, or 3/4 for taller muffins but the yield will be smaller. I use a 1/3 measuring cup to fill the cups.
11) Bake at 350 for 12 to 15 minutes or until firm and browning starts on top.
12) Remove from pan and place on a cooling rack for at least 5 minutes until they cool so they don't stick to the paper and serve.

# Protein Breakfast Scramble

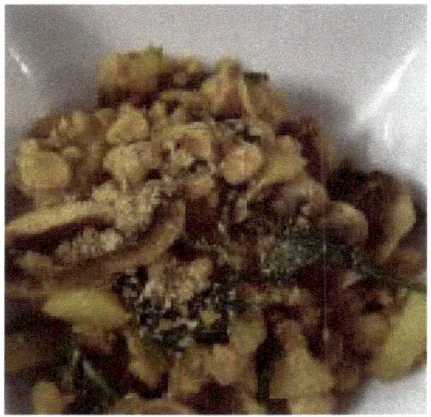

Grain free, high protein breakfast
Total Time: 10 mins
Servings: 4

Ingredients
- 2 cups cooked chickpeas
- 1/2 cup diced onion
- 1 peeled and diced squash
- 1 clove garlic, minced
- 5 washed and sliced mushrooms
- 1/2 lemon, juiced
- 1 handful spinach
- 1 Tbsp turmeric
- 1 Tbsp grated ginger
- 1 Tbsp nutritional yeast
- 1 cup vegetable broth
- 1 Tbsp cayenne pepper
- salt & pepper to taste

Instructions
1) Heat pan over high heat.
2) Add diced onions and stir continuously until translucent, about 1 minute.

3) Add garlic and mushrooms and continue to stir until it starts to stick to the pan, 1 more minute.
4) Add just enough vegetable broth to keep it from sticking.
5) Toss in squash, turmeric, salt, pepper, and cayenne, if using.
6) Continue to stir for about 1 minute.
7) Grate ginger over top and pour in the remaining vegetable broth.
8) Toss in spinach and cook until it starts to wilt, stirring occasionally.
9) Finish by squeezing juice of 1/2 lemon over the top.
10) Stir and serve with sprinkled nutritional yeast.

# Chocolate Cashew Vegan Pudding

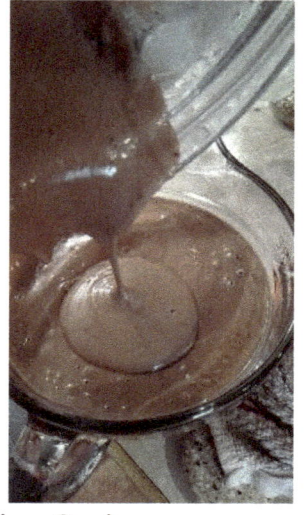 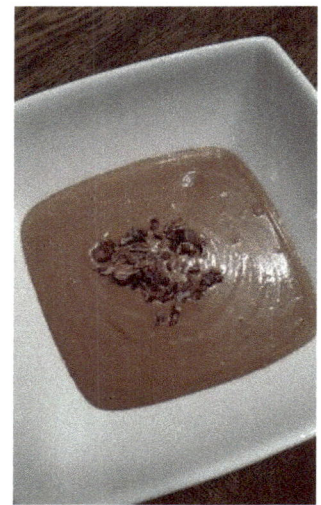

Prep Time 8 mins
Cool in refrigerator to set 4 hrs
Total Time: 4 hrs 8 mins
Servings: 5

Equipment
- Vitamix or other high-speed blender

Ingredients
- 2 ½ cups almond milk
- 1 cup cashews, unsalted
- 1 tbsp chia seeds
- 1 tsp vanilla
- 1 tbsp arrowroot
- 2 tbsp raw sugar, optional
- 1 tbsp cacao powder
- 1/4 cup cacao nibs sweetened optional
- 8 medjool dates, take out seeds
- 1 tsp nutmeg freshly grated

Instructions

264

1) Add all ingredients in high-speed blender.
2) Blend for 2 to 3 minutes or until smooth.
3) Add a tablespoon of almond milk or a little more if it's too thick or has a grainy texture.
4) Pour into a bowl, chill for at least 4 hours, and serve.

# Vegan waffles

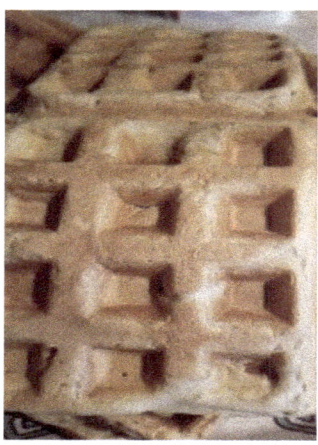

Prep Time: 5 mins
Total Time: 20 minutes
Servings: Approximately 18 waffles

Ingredients
- 1/2 cup almond flour
- 4 cups wheat or brown rice flour, for gluten free, or mix almond flour with wheat flour for flavor
- 1/4 cup vegan raw sugar
- 1 Tablespoon baking powder
- 1 Tablespoon vanilla
- 1 overripe smashed banana, peeled (use this instead of oil)
- Pinch of salt
- 4 cups plant-based milk - half cup extra may be necessary
- 1/4 cup egg replacer or arrowroot powder

Instructions
1) In a large mixing bowl, mix all ingredients until smooth. The mixture should be thick, but not too thick to pour. Add milk and stir until it's the right consistency.
2) Heat waffle maker to 400 degrees.

3) Pour in batter as per machine's instructions and cook for 2 to 4 minutes, depending on desired texture. If you're using almond flour, it will take longer to cook. Be patient.

# Lunch or Dinner
# Asian Soup

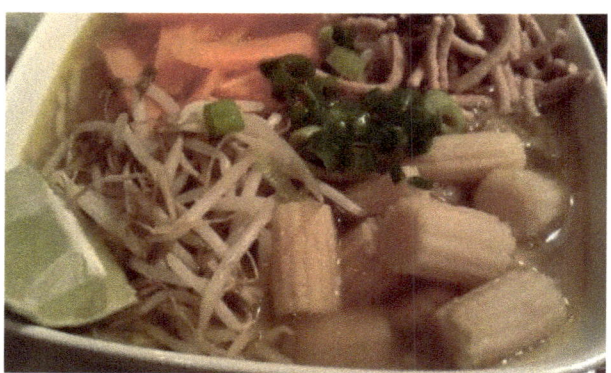

Prep Time: 20 mins
Total Time: 40 minutes
Servings: Approximately 4 servings

Ingredients
- 1 bag bean sprouts (about 3 cups)
- 1 package of noodles (any type of brown rice or whole grain noodle)
- 2 cloves of garlic, minced
- ¼ small onion, diced
- ½ tsp Turmeric
- 8 cups water
- 2 cups vegetable stock
- 2 carrots peeled and cut twice and then into thin pieces (depending on how crispy you like them)
- 1 can baby corn
- 1 tsp ginger, peeled and minced
- Crispy rice noodles (if you can find plant-based option)
- 1 lime
- 1 green onion, chopped
- ½ package Alfalfa Sprouts
- Any other Asian flavoring you like – to taste (I like soy sauce or teriyaki)

- Salt and pepper to taste

This recipe uses a lot of pans, but it's worth it!!!

Instructions
1) Heat non-stick soup pot over high heat.
2) Once hot, add minced garlic, diced onion, turmeric, ginger and Asian seasoning. Stir constantly until onions are translucent.
3) Add water, stock, or stock made with cubes, and bring to a boil.
4) Add salt and pepper to taste.
5) Reduce heat, cover, and simmer for 20 minutes on low flame.
6) In another pot, add about 10 cups of water and bring to a boil.
7) Drop in the bean sprouts and reduce heat slightly to cook for about five minutes.
8) In a medium sized pan, add 2 cups of water and carrots, bring to a boil and simmer over medium heat until cooked as desired.
9) In a small pan, heat the can of baby corn.
10) Wash and rinse alfalfa sprouts and drop them into soup pot a few minutes before soup is finished cooking...long enough to steam.
11) With a skimmer, pull bean sprouts out of boiling water and put into a bowl and set aside.
12) Drop the pasta into the still boiling (former bean sprout) water.
13) Once the pasta is cooked to desired tenderness, rinse and set aside in a bowl.
14) Wash and cut lime into wedges.
15) Chop the green onion, if you haven't already and set aside.
16) Once everything is cooked, turn off the heat to all of the pans, drain the corn and carrots and leave them in their pans.

17) Scoop 2 to 3 cups of soup into a bowl. The soup should just be the liquids, onion, garlic, ginger, and spices and the cooked alfalfa sprouts. Nothing else goes into the soup pot.

18) Now it's time to build your soup. Into the serving bowl that has your soup, add some of the pasta, carrots, bean sprouts, corn, and crispy noodles...add them separately. If you want to create a presentation, as in the picture, place the ingredients in separate areas of the bowl.

19) Squeeze a slice of lime over the top and add the lime wedge into the bowl to squeeze more as desired.

20) Top with the chopped green onions and add more salt and pepper if needed and serve.

# Black-eyed Pea and Quinoa Soup

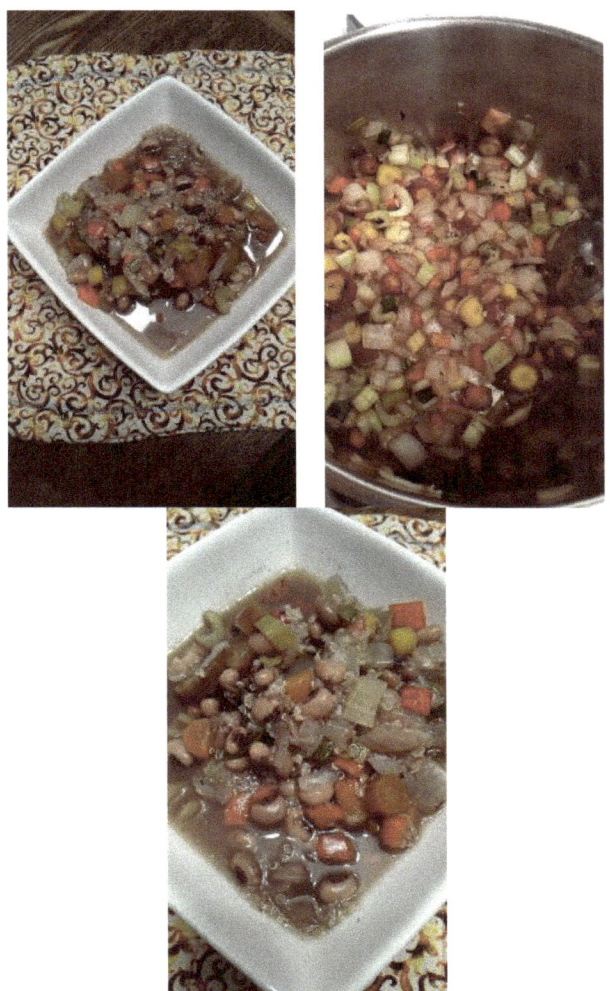

Ingredients
- 1 can black-eyed peas, drained
- 1 cup onion, cut small
- 2 cloves garlic, minced
- 4 carrots, cut small (I used rainbow carrots)
- 1/2 cup bell peppers, cut small
- 2 stalks celery, cut small
- 1 cup veggie stock

- Salt and pepper to taste
- 1/2 teaspoon eucalyptus, minced (optional)
- 1/2 teaspoon oregano
- 1/2 teaspoon rosemary
- 1 cup quinoa
- 6 to 8 cups of water

Instructions
1) Heat pan to high heat, add onions, garlic, celery, carrots, and bell peppers to hot pan, sauté, stirring constantly until onions are translucent. Add water by the spoonful if they start to stick to the pan.
2) Add the rest of the water, the blackened peas, seasonings and quinoa.
3) Turn the heat to medium and simmer until quinoa has opened.
4) Remove from heat and serve.

# Bok Choy Burritos

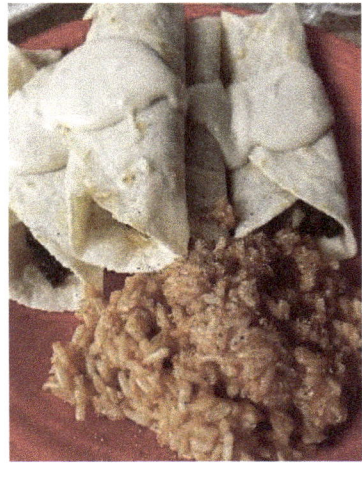
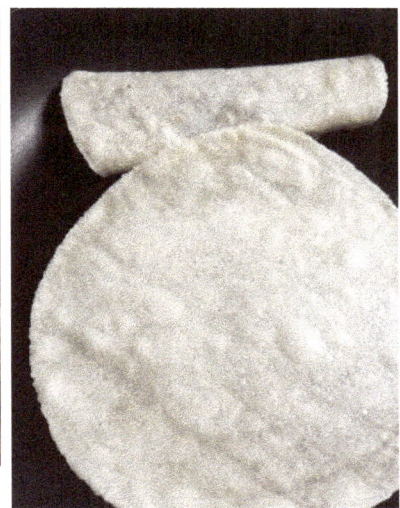

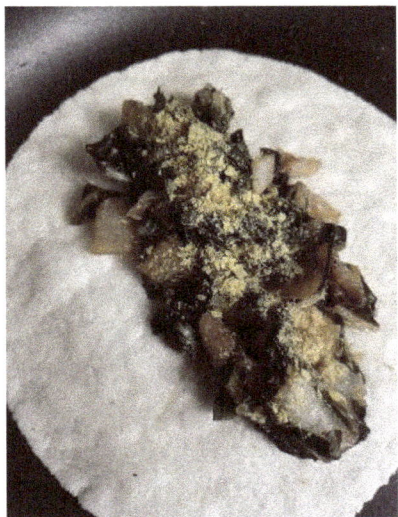

Makes 6 – 8 burritos
Prep time: 10 minutes
Cook time: 20 minutes

See Maria's Spanish Rice Recipe for the rice.
Ingredients

- 1 head of bok choy or napa cabbage (I actually prefer to use the napa if I can find it.)
- 2 cloves minced garlic
- ¼ cup teriyaki sauce
- 1/4 cup nutritional yeast
- 6 to 8 tortillas - pictured are almond flour tortillas
- Pepper to taste (the teriyaki sauce is salty, so I don't usually add more salt)
- Cashew cream and salsa for topping

Instructions
1) Wash and chop or shred the cabbage into small pieces. I do about 2 by 2 inches.
2) Add cabbage to pan or wok heated over medium fire.
3) Add garlic and sauce.
4) Cover and reduce heat. The cabbage will release water and simmer down. Let simmer until cabbage is a meaty texture. Stir occasionally and drain excess water if necessary.
5) Remove from heat and in a separate pan, heat one side of tortilla for about 30 seconds over low heat.
6) Flip tortilla and spoon in cabbage filling (about 2 Tablespoons) and top with desired amount of nutritional yeast.
7) Fold tortilla and let it sit in pan for about 30 seconds to get crispy.
8) Continue with the next tortilla until all the cabbage is used.
9) Top with salsa and cashew cream.

# Butternut Squash Soup

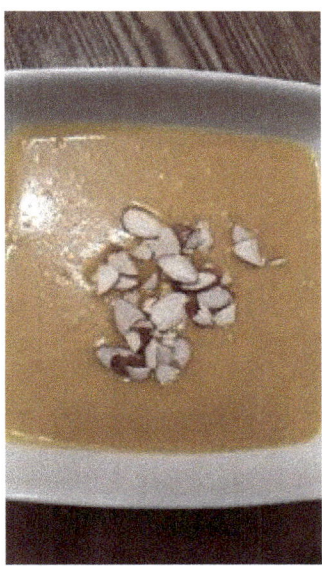

Ingredients
- 1 medium butternut squash, peeled and cut into cubes
- 4 cups vegetable stock
- 1 medium onion, sliced
- 2 cups almond or any nut milk
- 1/2 teaspoon nutmeg
- 1 tablespoon cinnamon
- 1/2 teaspoon sweet paprika
- 1 teaspoon paprika
- Pumpkin seeds or chopped cashews or almonds for topping
- Salt and pepper to taste

Instructions
1) Peel and cut butternut squash and onion.
2) Heat pan to high heat until very hot.
3) Add onion slices, stirring constantly until translucent.

4) Add butternut squash and sauté for about 2 minutes, stirring constantly.
5) Add vegetable stock and everything else, except the milk.
6) Stir, reduce heat to medium and simmer for about 15 minutes or until squash is tender.
7) Add milk and stir. Simmer for an additional 5 minutes.
8) Pour soup into high-speed blender in batches if necessary and blend until smooth.
9) Return soup to the pan and taste. Add necessary salt, pepper, or paprika to taste.
10) If the soup is too thin, blend cashews or a potato with it until desired consistency. If soup is too thick, add water.
11) Serve hot, topping with desired nut or seed.

# Cabbage Rolls

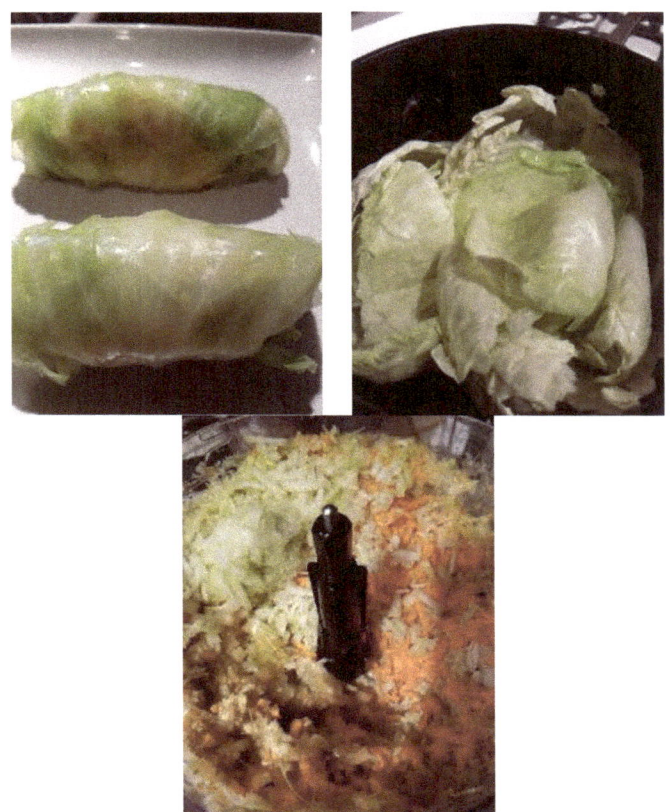

Makes 12 to 14 rolls
Ingredients

- 1 head cabbage
- 1/2 cup onion
- 4 carrots
- 2 - 15 ounce cans garbanzo beans, drained
- 3 celery stalks
- 1/2 cup cashews
- 1/4 teaspoon smoked paprika
- 1 to 2 tablespoons dill, to taste
- 1 teaspoon garlic powder
- 1 teaspoon onion powder

277

- •     2 tablespoons lemon pepper
- •     Juice of a lemon
- •     Salt and pepper to taste

Instructions
1) Boil large pot of salted water for cabbage leaves.
2) Wash and peel leaves from cabbage, try not to tear.
3) Put cabbage leaves in boiling water for about 5 minutes or until desired tenderness. Stir carefully with tongs to cook evenly. Remove promptly and place on tray or plate to cool.
4) In a food processor, add garbanzo beans, cashews, and spices. Process until smooth.
5) Take out bottom blade and replace with shredding blade.
6) Shred carrots, celery, and onions on top of mixture.
7) Remove blade and stir to mix well.
8) Lay out cabbage leaves one at a time. Put in approximately 2 tablespoons of filling in narrow end, fold in sides, and roll until secure.

# Cabbage Soup

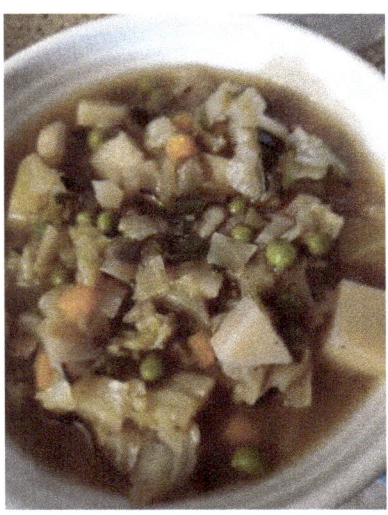

Makes 6 servings
Prep time: 10 minutes
Cook time: 50 minutes

Ingredients
- 3 large carrots (sliced)
- 1 cup dry chickpeas or garbanzo beans (rinsed)
- ½ onion, chopped
- 2 cloves minced garlic
- ½ head of cabbage
- 2 stalks celery, chopped
- 1 package alfalfa sprouts
- 4 cups vegetable stock
- 2 cups water (add more if needed as chickpeas cook and absorb water
- ½ teaspoon turmeric
- Salt & pepper to taste

Instructions
1) Heat large pot over medium heat.

279

2) Immediately add chopped onion, celery, and carrots.
3) Cook over medium heat, stirring occasionally for about 5 minutes.
4) Add vegetable stock, water, chickpeas, garlic, cabbage, turmeric, and salt and pepper.
5) Bring to a boil.
6) Reduce heat to medium and simmer for approximately 40 minutes or until chickpeas are almost tender.
7) Add alfalfa sprouts for last five minutes.
8) Serve once chickpeas are tender.

# Pea Protein Carrot Soup

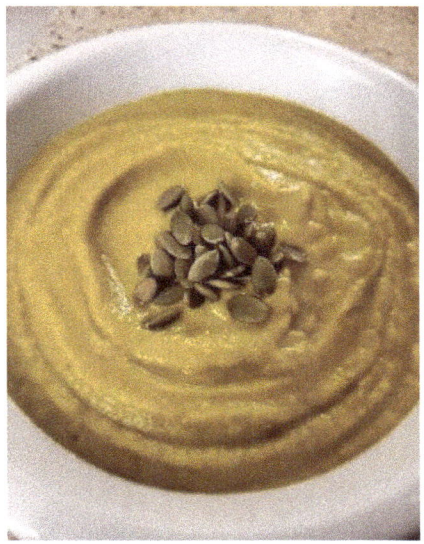

Ingredients
- 1/2 onion, diced
- 2 cloves garlic, peeled
- 2 tablespoons white wine
- 3 cups carrots, peeled and chopped into approximately 1 inch pieces
- 1 cup frozen peas
- 1 cup vegetable stock
- 3 to 4 cups water, to desired texture
- 1 cup cashews
- 1 dash tabasco sauce
- Salt and pepper to taste

Instructions
1) Heat metal pan until hot
2) Add onions and garlic and stir constantly until onions are translucent
3) Deglaze pan with white wine, stir 1 minute
4) Add carrots and stir 2 minutes
5) Add vegetable stock and salt and pepper
6) Add peas and enough water to cover the mixture.

7) Turn down heat and simmer until peas are tender.
8) In a high-speed blender, add cashews and tabasco sauce
9) Pour carrot mixture into blender and blend on high speed until you reach desired texture, adding water as necessary.
10) Pour soup back into pan and check flavor. Add more salt and pepper as necessary and add your favorite plant-based milk if you like it creamy.
11) Top with pumpkin seeds or your favorite garnish

# Southwest Bowl

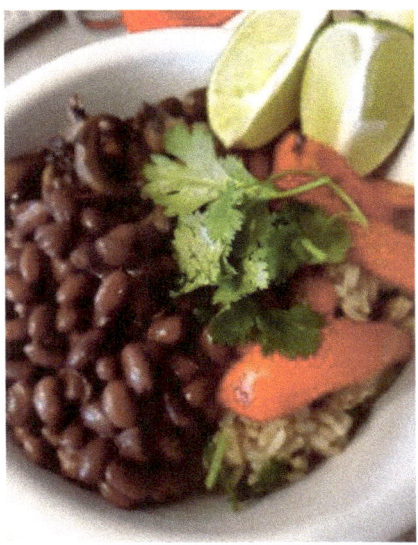

Prep Time: 5 mins
Total Time: 20 minutes
Servings: 2

Ingredients
- 4 cups cooked brown rice – cooking time will increase if not using leftover or pre-cooked rice
- 1 can black beans
- ½ cup drunken mushrooms (approx. 8 mushrooms) (see recipe or look below in the instructions)
- 1 red bell pepper
- 1 clove of garlic
- ½ cup diced onion
- 1 tsp cumin
- 1 tsp basil
- 2 tbsp nutritional yeast
- ½ cup red wine or vegetable stock
- ½ cup cilantro, cut into 2-inch pieces, reserve a couple of sprigs to top the dish
- 1 lime, sliced into quarter pieces
- Salt and pepper to taste

Instructions
1) Wash and slice approx. 8 mushrooms.
2) Wash and slice bell pepper.
3) Dice onion.
4) Wash and cut cilantro.
5) Sauté onion and garlic in medium sized pan (big enough to hold rice) until translucent, about 1 minute stirring constantly so it doesn't stick. (See Chef Secrets chapter to learn how to sauté onion.) Deglaze the pan with wine or vegetable stock.
6) Add rice, cumin, basil, nutritional yeast, and cilantro to the onion and garlic blend. Add salt and pepper to taste. Turn the heat down to low and stir occasionally, add ¼ cup of water if necessary to keep the rice from sticking to the pan.
7) Drunken mushroom recipe --- Add mushrooms to a small pan with salt and pepper on medium heat. Stir occasionally. When the mushrooms start to release their juices, add about ¼ cup of red wine and reduce to simmer, stirring occasionally, until mushrooms reach the desired texture. Remove from heat and set aside in a small bowl. You can use vegetable stock instead of wine. The flavor won't be as savory, but it can be used as a substitute.
8) Heat the black beans per the instructions on can. You can put them in a microwave safe bowl and heat in the microwave for 2 minutes or until they come to a boil if you don't want to heat them on the stove.
9) In the pan you used for the mushrooms, add the bell pepper slices. Cook on medium heat, stirring occasionally until desired texture. Remove from heat and set aside.
10) Assemble the bowl by putting half the rice in the bowl and add the pepper, mushrooms, black beans, and cilantro sprigs. Top with the juice of half the lime. Serve.

# SPICY CHILI

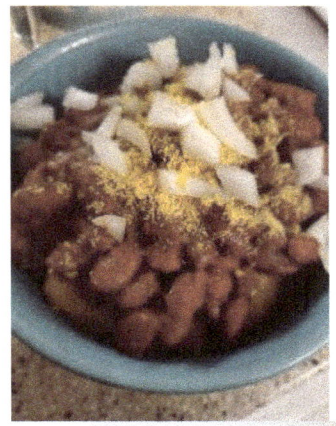

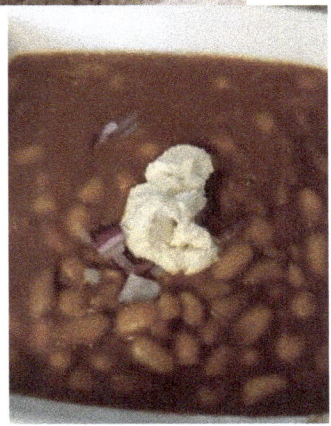

Prep Time: 5 mins
Total Time: 10 minutes
Servings: 2

Ingredients
- 6 to 10 cups of beans with juice (I used leftover pinto and mix them with red kidney or black beans)
- 1 small can tomato paste
- 1/4 onion, chopped small
- 1/4 cup beer or red wine
- 1/4 cup chili powder

- 1 dash of vegan Worcestershire sauce
- 2 cloves minced garlic
- 1 TB ground cumin
- 1 TB dried oregano
- 1 TB dried basil
- 1 teaspoon paprika
- 1 TB sugar
- Salt and Pepper to taste

Instructions
1) Mix all of the ingredients into medium sized pot under high heat and bring to boil.
2) Reduce heat to simmer until desired consistency or until onions are to desired tenderness - about 15 minutes.
3) Serve over plant-based crackers, chips, or in a tortilla.
4) Top with onion and nutritional yeast, if desired. I love it topped with sour cream.

# Spinach and Squash Enchiladas

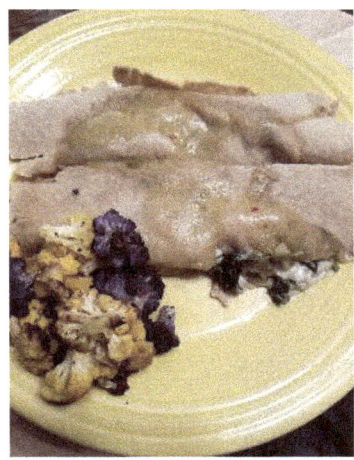
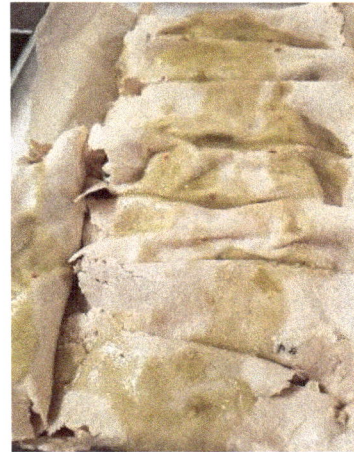

Ingredients
- 10 to 12 wheat tortillas
- 3 medium yellow squash, peeled and diced
- 4 cups spinach
- 1 small onion, diced
- 1green bell pepper, diced
- 2 cans el Paso green chili sauce
- 2 cups cashews
- 3 to 4 cups water
- 1/4 cup nutritional yeast

Instructions
1) Preheat oven to 350.
2) Line 1 to 2 casserole dishes with parchment paper.
3) In a hot large skillet, sauté squash, onion, and bell pepper until onions are translucent, stirring constantly. If the vegetables stick to the pan, add water by the tablespoon.
4) Stir in spinach and sauté for 2 to 3 minutes, until wilted.
5) Stir in 1 can of green chili sauce and salt and pepper to taste, reduce heat to a simmer.

287

6) In a high-speed blender, blend cashews, nutritional yeast, and water, starting with 3 cups of water and adding more as necessary for desired consistency. It should be a creamy thick sauce.

7) Add cashew cream to the vegetable mixture by the tablespoon and stir, simmer until desired texture. Put leftover cashew cream, if any, in the refrigerator for up to one week and use as a dip, thickener, or sour cream replacement.

8) Scoop 2 to 3 tablespoons of vegetable mixture into tortillas and roll into enchilada shape.

9) Place enchiladas into prepared casserole dishes and pour 1 can of green chili sauce over the top.

10) Bake at 350 for 15 to 20 minutes, or until tortillas are slightly browned.

# Hawaiian Barbeque Bowl

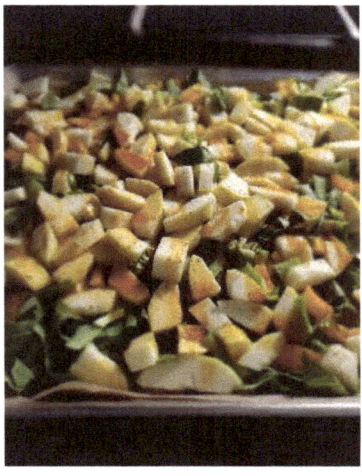 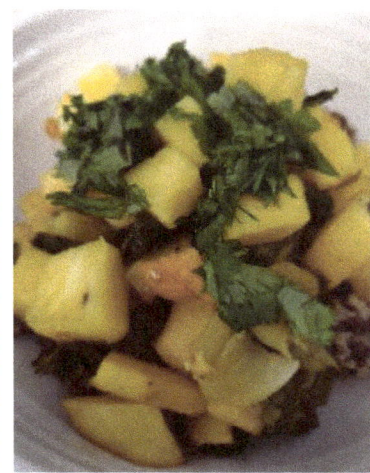

Prep Time: 10 mins
Total Time: 20 minutes
Servings: 4

Ingredients
- 4 zucchini peeled and sliced
- 2 cups baby bok choy chopped
- 1 tsp ginger grated
- 2 bell pepper diced
- 1 cup pineapple cubed
- 1/4 cup barbeque sauce
- 1/4 cup cilantro chopped

Instructions
1) Preheat oven to 425 and line a baking pan with parchment paper.
2) Prepare the ingredients by chopping and dicing and place the zucchini, bok choy, and bell pepper on the baking pan. Add salt and pepper and drizzle with barbeque sauce.
3) Cover with aluminum foil and cook for 10 minutes.
4) While the vegetables are cooking, prepare quinoa or farrow for the base of the dish as per instructions on

the package and cube the pineapple and chop the cilantro.

5) Remove cover from the vegetables, drizzle with water, and cook an additional 10 minutes or until the zucchini is tender.

6) Once the zucchini is cooked, remove the baking pan from the oven and grate fresh ginger over the top. Add quinoa or farrow to your plate. Top with the cooked zucchini mixture, pineapple, and cilantro and serve.

# Vegan Beer Hot Dogs

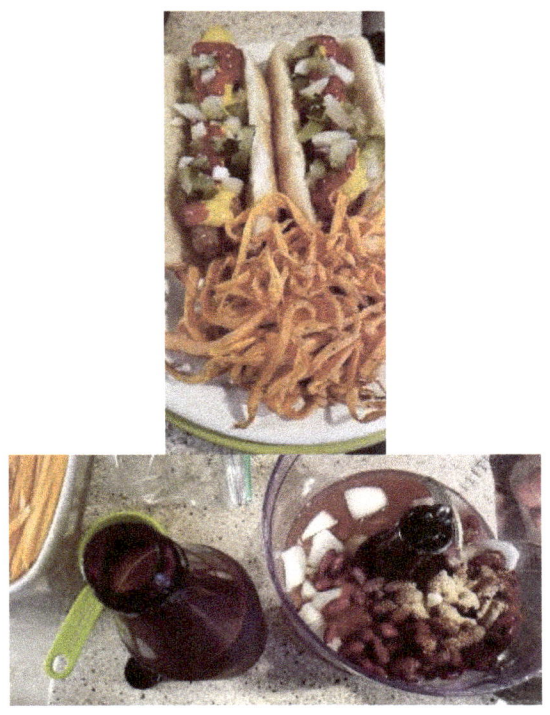

Yield 10 to 12 hot dogs
Time: 50 minutes

Ingredients
- 1 can or equivalent chickpeas, drained
- 1 can or equivalent red kidney beans, drained
- 1/2 white or yellow onion
- 2 cloves garlic
- 1/4 cup ketchup
- 1/4 cup mustard
- 2 tablespoons smoked paprika
- 2 tablespoons liquid smoke
- 1 tablespoon garlic powder
- 1/2 cup water
- 1/4 cup vegan beer

- Salt and pepper to taste
- 1 cup Chipotle peppers in sauce for spicy version
- Dry ingredients
- 1/2 cup vital wheat gluten
- 1 cup rolled oats
- 2 to 3 cups chickpea flour
- 1 tablespoon arrowroot
- 1/2 cup nutritional yeast

Instructions

1) Set up a large pot for steaming, with the water level just below the grate. Bring to a boil.
2) In a food processor, add all ingredients except for Chipotle and dry ingredients. Mix well.
3) Cut aluminum foil and parchment pa per into strips large enough to roll around your desired hot dog size with enough foil to roll around at least twice and fold up at the ends. I use approximately 12" by 6" strips, but they don't have to be precise. I prep these by putting the parchment paper on top of each foil strip in a stack of parchment, foil, parchment, foil, and so on.
4) In a large mixing bowl, add your dry ingredients and stir with a spoon or fork just to blend.
5) Add the mixture from the food processor to the dry ingredients and mix by hand for a couple of minutes. If it's too wet, add more chickpea flour. If it's too dry, add a little bit of water at a time. It should be slightly sticky and not too dry, but hold its shape.
6) Once the dough is the desired consistency, roll it into 10 to 12 even balls.
7) One at a time, roll the balls between your hands and create an oblong, hot dog shape of your desired size.
8) Starting at the end of a piece of parchment paper, roll the hot dog into the paper and then roll it into the foil, folding up the ends. Do each hot dog the same way until each is in a foil wrapper.
9) Stack the hot dogs into the steamer side by side, putting each layer in the opposite direction to allow

steam to rise. Leave some room between each hot dog.

10) Put a lid on the steamer and steam for about 20 minutes, checking the water level 2 or 3 times and adding more as necessary. Make sure the water line stays below the foil packs.

11) Remove and heat in a non-stick skillet for about 2 minutes, rolling them in the pan to heat evenly. If you're making a spicy version, add Chipotle sauce at the ratio of 2 tablespoons per hot dog while heating.

12) Serve with your favorite toppings.

# Chickpea Meatballs

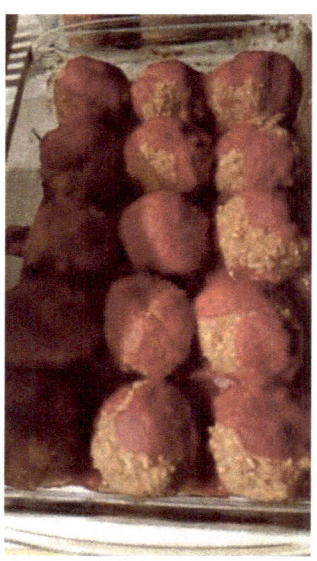

Makes approximately 20 balls

Ingredients
- 2 cans organic chickpeas or about 32 ounces of cooked chickpeas (drained)
- 2 cans organic tomato sauce (12 ounce)
- 2 to 3 cups rolled oats
- 2 cups cooked brown rice (measured at 2 cups before cooked)
- 3 tablespoons egg replacer or arrowroot
- 1/2 teaspoon oregano
- ½ teaspoon basil
- ½ teaspoon thyme
- Salt and pepper to taste

Instructions
1) Cook rice as per instructions on package
2) Preheat oven to 400 degrees Fahrenheit

3) Add chickpeas to food processor and blend for about 2 minutes or until smooth.
4) Add egg replacer or arrowroot, salt, pepper, seasonings, and 1 can of tomato sauce to food processor. Turn on for 2 minutes.
5) Add rice to food processor and pulse, just until it's mixed in.
6) Remove the blade from the processor and stir in 2 cups of oats until the mixture is no longer soggy and will form into a ball. If needed, add more oats until the mixture sticks together without being sticky.
7) Form into balls and place in baking dish, leaving room in between for scooping out the balls.
8) Pour other can of tomato sauce over the balls.
9) Bake for 20 minutes or until cooked through.
10) Serve with pasta, on the side of mashed potatoes and green beans, or on bread as a sandwich.

# Chickpea Patties

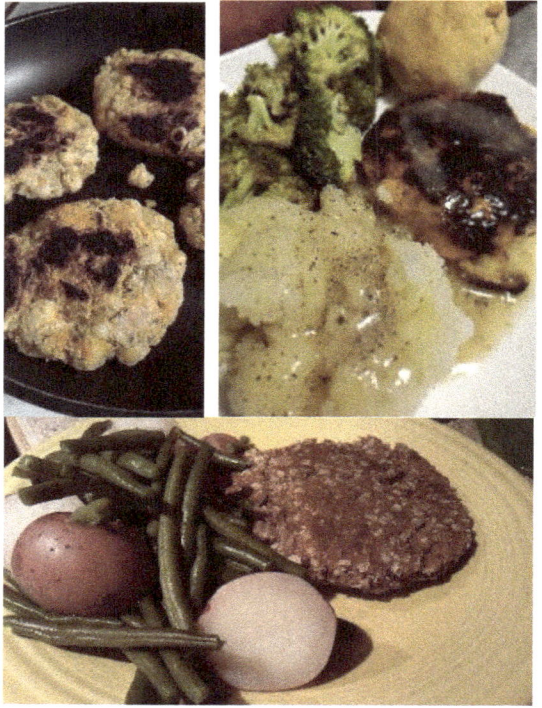

Makes approximately 8 patties, depending on size.

Ingredients
    You can use lentils, chickpeas, or black beans.

If you want to use half the squash and save half after baking it, you can use the squash for a puree for butternut squash risotto or as a base for other recipes.

- 1 can or approximately 16 ounces lentils, mostly drained (or your choice of legumes)
- 1 butternut squash, peeled and diced into 1-inch cubes

296

- 1 cup oatmeal or almond flour
- 1 tablespoon egg replacer or tapioca flour or arrowroot
- 1 teaspoon garlic powder
- 1 tablespoon Cajun seasoning or mixture of paprika, cayenne pepper, onion powder, and thyme
- 2 tablespoons nutritional yeast
- Dash of dried oregano
- 1 tablespoon lemon pepper
- 2 tablespoons vegetable stock
- Salt and pepper

Instructions
1) Heat oven to 425.
2) Peel butternut squash and dice.
3) Spread squash onto baking sheet with parchment paper and coat with salt, pepper, lemon pepper, and vegetable stock.
4) Cook squash for approximately 25 to 30 minutes in a 425-degree oven or until tender.
5) Put everything except almond flour or oatmeal into food processor until blended. If you like chunky patties, I use a potato masher or dough cutter in a bowl and blend and mash by hand.
6) Add flour or oatmeal and 1 tablespoon at a time of water if necessary to make patties stick together.
7) Put nonstick frying pan on stove over high heat.
8) With your hands, create a ball with the mixture, then flatten into patty. Continue, makes about 8 patties.
9) Heat frying pan until pan is very hot. A sprinkle of water should turn into a mercury ball.
10) Fry patties for about 3 to 4 minutes on each side until brown. If the patties start to burn, turn the heat down to medium once you've browned both sides.
11) Top with A1 or your favorite sauce or gravy.
12) If you want to make a quick version, don't use butternut squash and just double the amount of legumes.

# Irish Colcannon

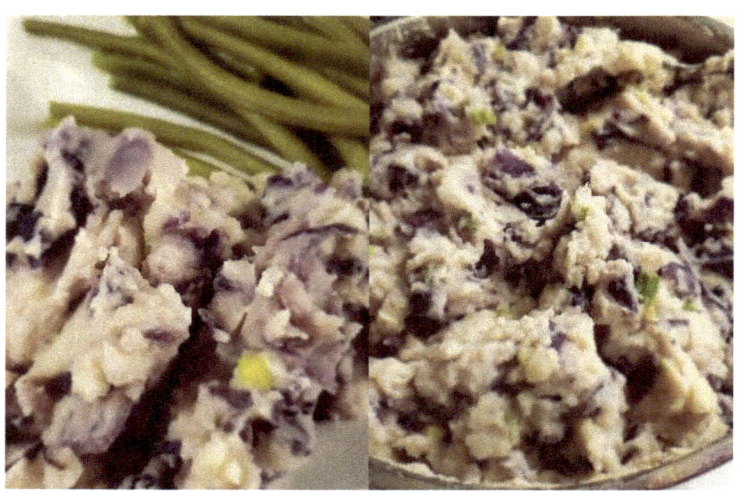

Prep Time 10 mins
Cook Time: 20 mins
Servings: 6

Ingredients
- 1 small head of cabbage, washed and shredded
- 4 large potatoes, peeled and diced
- 8 green onions, washed and diced
- 1 cup cashews
- 1 lime
- 1 cup water
- 5 cups vegetable stock
- Salt
- Pepper
- Fresh grated nutmeg

Directions
1) Boil potatoes in large pan of water until tender.
2) While potatoes are boiling, heat saucepan until hot. Add cabbage and salt and pepper and stir

occasionally so it doesn't burn. Turn down heat and stir every few minutes. Cook until tender.

3) Put cashews, juice of 1 lime, salt, pepper, and 1 cup of water in blender. Blend on high until creamy. Add more water, if necessary, by tablespoon. Set aside.

4) Heat a small saucepan until hot, add onions and sauté', stirring constantly for 2 minutes. Add vegetable stock if necessary to keep from burning. Turn down heat to low.

5) Pour cashew cream into pan with onions. Add 4 cups vegetable stock and stir. Cook for 2 minutes over low heat. Set aside.

6) Drain and mash potatoes. Add 1 cup vegetable stock.

7) Pour mashed potatoes and cabbage into cashew cream. Cook over low heat until fully mixed. Add salt and pepper to taste. Garnish with fresh ground nutmeg.

# Mushroom Bisque

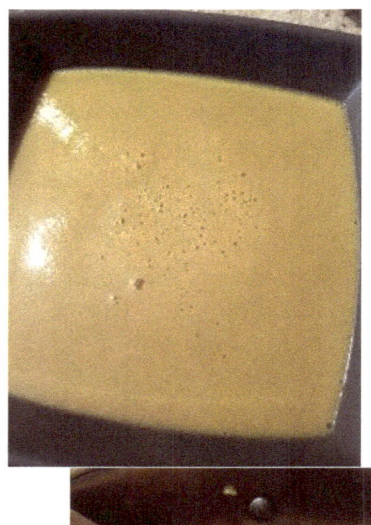

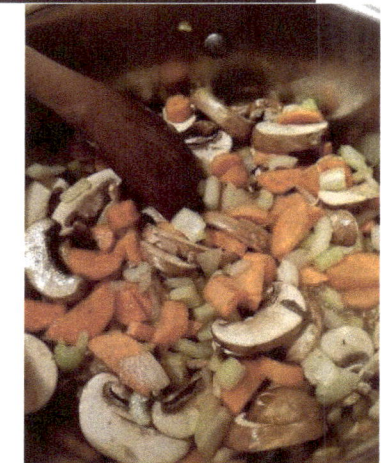

Ingredients

- 1 pound mushrooms (about 12), washed and sliced
- 2 carrots, sliced
- 4 stalks celery, sliced
- 1 small onion, diced
- 2 cloves of garlic, peeled, no need to mince

- 8 cups vegetable stock or water with 1 veggie bouillon cube
- 1 tsp rosemary
- 1 tsp basil
- 1 tsp thyme
- Salt and pepper to taste
- 1 bay leaf
- 2 tablespoons flour
- 1 cup cashews
- 1 to 2 cups water, for cashews
- Pumpkin seeds for topping

Instructions

1) In a hot pan, add mushrooms, carrots, celery, onion, and garlic. Stir constantly until the onions are translucent. If the vegetables start to stick to the pan, add water by 1 tablespoon at a time.
2) Once the onions are translucent, add the water or vegetable stock. Add spices and bay leaf.
3) Turn down heat and simmer for 20 minutes.
4) In a high-speed blender, add cashews and water for cashews. Blend until smooth, adding more water as necessary.
5) After base has simmered, remove bay leaf.
6) Heat sauté pan to high heat. Scoop out 2 cups of base soup and add to sauté pan. Add flour and, stirring constantly, make a roux. Add more base soup as necessary to create a smooth roux. For those not from the south, a roux is gravy. ☺
7) Add roux to base soup and stir.
8) In batches, add soup to cashew mix in blender. Blend on high speed until smooth and pour into large bowl and stir batches together.

# Creamy Mushroom Soup

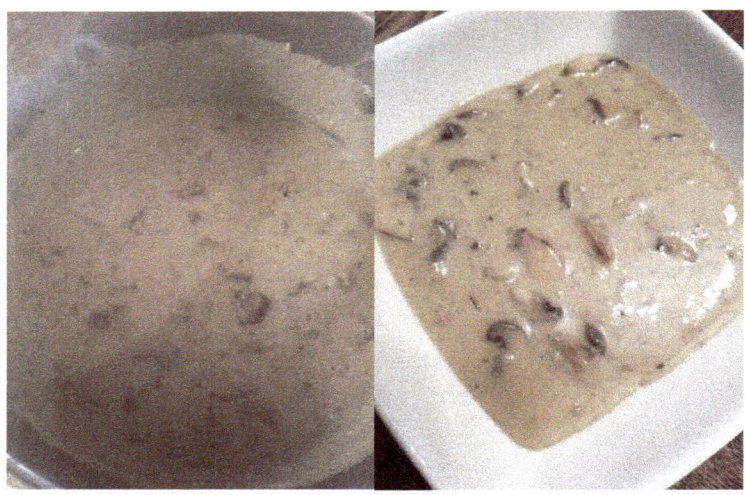

15 minutes
2 to 3 servings

Ingredients
- 1/2 onion, diced
- 6 large mushrooms or 2 cups, chopped
- 5 cloves garlic, minced
- 2 cups vegetable stock
- 4 to 6 cups almond milk
- 1 tablespoon dried oregano
- 1 veggie bouillon cube or 2 cups of vegetable stock and only 4 cups of almond milk
- 2 to 3 tablespoons wheat flour
- Dash of nutmeg
- Salt and pepper to taste

Instructions
1) Heat non-reactive (metal) pan on high heat until water evaporates in pan.

2) Add mushrooms, onions, and garlic and stir constantly until onions are translucent, about 3 minutes.
3) Add seasonings and 1 tablespoon flour, coating mixture.
4) Pour in stock and 1 more tablespoon of flour and whisk, bring to a boil and whisk constantly while adding almond milk.
5) Turn down heat to medium and let thicken.
6) Add bouillon cube or vegetable stock and nutmeg.
7) Add more almond milk or flour if necessary to thicken to desired consistency, about 10 minutes. Stir frequently.
8) Use an immersion blender or add soup to a blender if you don't want chunks.

# Creamy Vegan Penne Pasta with Peas

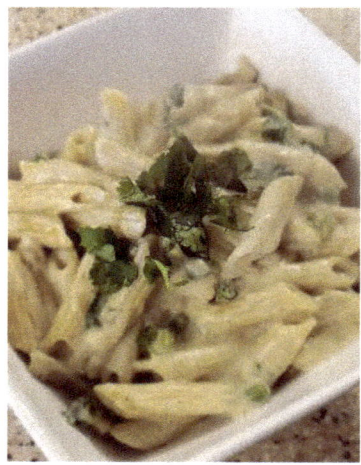 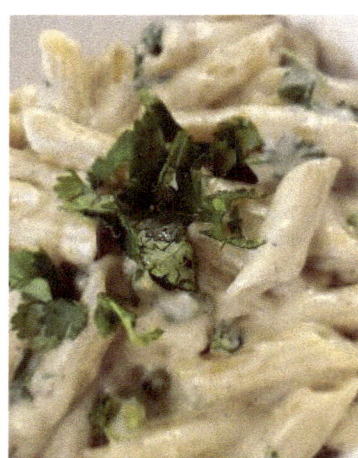

Prep Time: 5 mins
Cook Time: 20 mins
Servings: 6

Ingredients
- 1 package penne pasta, your favorite vegan brand
- 1/2 bag frozen peas
- 1/2 onion diced
- 2 tbsp white wine
- 2 tbsp flour, I use wheat, but you can use almond
- 2 cups water or more if needed to created base sauce
- 1 tbsp oregano
- 1 tbsp basil
- 1 tbsp lemon pepper
- 1 tbsp vegan Worcestershire sauce

- 1 salt & pepper to taste
- 1 clove garlic minced
- 1 tbsp nutritional yeast
- 2 cups cashews
- 1 cup water for cashews Add more if needed to get creamy consistency
- 1/4 cup cilantro chopped and added as a garnish, if desired

Instructions
1) Bring a pot of water to boil and add salt
2) Dice onions and prepare ingredients because this recipe will move quickly and you'll want everything prepped to go.
3) Make slurry with one cup of the water, flour, and seasonings
4) Bring metal skillet to high heat, hot enough to create a mercury ball with a drop of water
5) Drop pasta and peas into the boiling water and cook to desired tenderness
6) Add onions to the hot skillet and, stir constantly for about 1 minute or until translucent
7) Add wine to the onions and stir until wine evaporates
8) Pour your slurry into the skillet and using a whisk, stir constantly until it comes to a boil
9) Add the remaining ingredients to the skillet, including 1 cup of extra water
10) Using a whisk, continue to stir the sauce and add more water if needed
11) Drain the pasta and peas when done, but reserve 2 cups of drained water in a bowl
12) Turn down the heat on the sauce to a simmer
13) In a high-speed blender, add cashews and one cup of water. Blend on high until the cashews are creamy texture. Add more water if needed or more cashews if there is too much liquid.
14) Pour pasta and peas into the skillet with the sauce. Stir until covered.
15) Pour reserved pasta water into the skillet and then add the cashew cream. Stir

16) Adjust seasoning as necessary and garnish with additional nutritional yeast and chopped cilantro, if desired.

# POTATO AND BLACK BEAN HASH

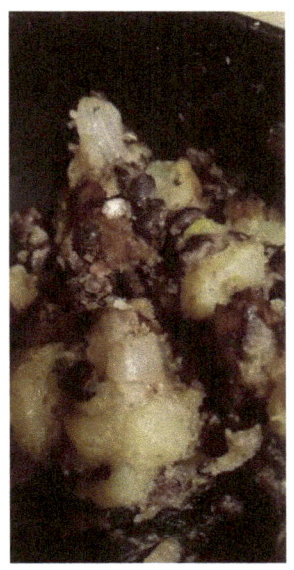
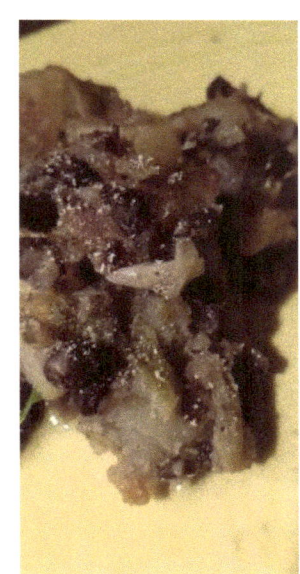

Ingredients

- 4 large potatoes or approximately two pounds, peeled and cut into cubes
- 1 can of black beans, drained and rinsed. I used about 2 pounds of potatoes, so I used the large can of beans.
- 1 small can of diced green chilis
- 1/2 onion diced, or less, if making a small batch
- Salt and pepper to taste
- Nutritional yeast to taste, I used 1/2 cup
- Oregano to taste

Instructions
1) Heat nonstick skillet until hot.
2) Add potatoes and onions and seasonings.

3) Cover with a lid and cook on medium, tossing occasionally to keep from burning and cook evenly.
4) When close to desired tenderness turn heat to low and add beans and chilis.
5) Taste and add any additional seasoning desired.
6) Heat until warmed through and serve.

# Maria's Spanish Rice

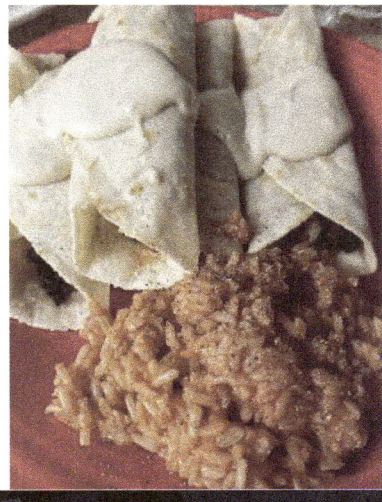

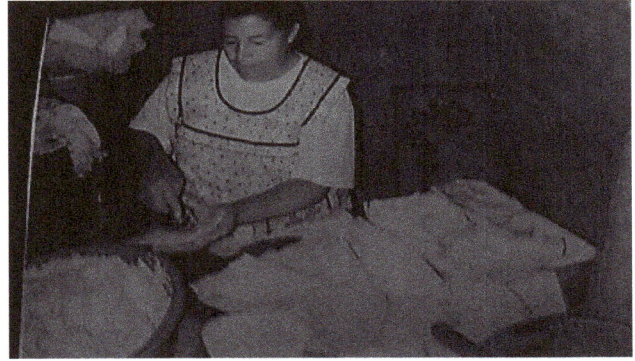

This is my mother-in-law's recipe, minus oil.

The picture shows Maria in her kitchen in Mexico, making Christmas tamales.

Maria's rice recipe

Makes 6 – 8 servings
Prep time: 10 minutes
Cook time: 40 minutes to 1 hour

Ingredients

- • 1 Can tomato Sauce or crushed tomatoes, at least 8 oz
- • 1 small can of tomato paste (if you like more acidity)
- • 1 cup of long grain brown rice
- • 2 cloves of garlic
- • 1 tablespoon of salt
- • ¼ cup onion, diced
- • 1 can of whole corn (optional)
- • 4 ¼ cup water

Instructions

1) The secret to my mother-in-law's rice is to get the oil hot. I don't use oil, so I get the pan hot.
2) Prepare your ingredients before you heat the pan.
3) Chop the onion, mince the garlic, and get your tomato sauce and paste (if you're using paste) ready. Also, put your cup of water on the counter. Have everything prepared, because once you start cooking, you won't have time to get anything else.
4) Mince the garlic with a mortar and pestle. I put the salt in the bottom and then ¼ cup of the water and then I cut the garlic into small pieces and mince it in there. I've tried it other ways, but mincing the garlic with the salt adds an authentic flavor to the soup or rice.
5) Sprinkle water into the pan and if it forms a mercury ball, it's ready.
6) Pour in the rice and minced onions and stir constantly until the onions are translucent and a golden-brown color. This takes about 5 minutes.
7) Immediately pour in the minced garlic/salt mixture, the tomato sauce, tomato paste, water, and corn, if you're using it.
8) Don't stir...just add more water as needed and cook until the rice is tender.
9) When using brown rice, it takes about 30 to 40 minutes of cooking and then cover it for about 10 minutes to soften.

# Red Beans and Cauliflower Rice with a Balsamic Reduction

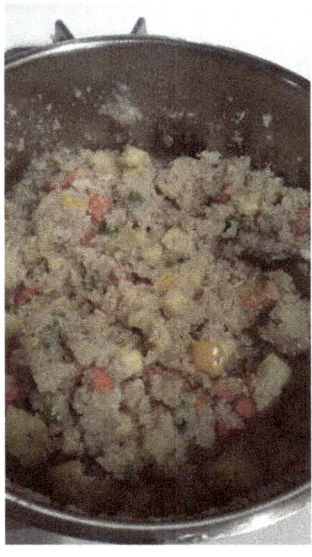 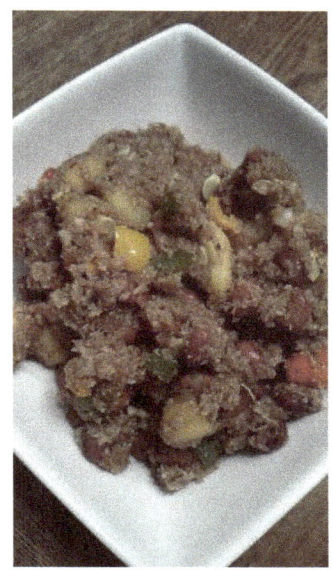

Prep Time: 10 mins
Cook Time: 30 mins
Servings: 4

Ingredients
- 2 cups red beans, cooked
- 1 head cauliflower
- 1 yellow squash, diced into 2 inch cubes
- 1/2 cup assorted bell peppers, diced small
- 2 cups balsamic vinegar
- 1 1/2 tablespoon cajun seasoning
- 1 tablespoon lemon pepper
- 1/2 tablespoon onion powder
- 2 cups vegetable stock.

Instructions
1) Cut cauliflower into small pieces and put in food processor on pulse, just until the texture is consistent. Don't over process.

2) Using a non-reactive pan, pour in balsamic vinegar and bring to a boil, stirring occasionally. Turn down heat to a low boil. Continue to cook while you prepare the "rice" for about 15 to 20 minutes, or until the balsamic is reduced by half. Check it continually in the last 10 minutes to make sure it doesn't burn. When it coats the spoon, it's finished.

3) In a hot pan, add the bell peppers and squash and sauté until the peppers are soft. Add vegetable stock by the spoonful to the pan if they start to stick and stir continuously, about 3 minutes.

4) Add cauliflower and about 1/2 cup vegetable stock and continue stirring until the cauliflower is browned.

5) Pour in the rest of the stock and add all of the seasonings and salt and pepper to taste.

6) Turn down the heat to low, add the beans, and cook for an additional 2 to 3 minutes until the mixture absorbs the stock.

7) If the balsamic reduction has hardened, heat it over low heat, stirring constantly and add more balsamic if necessary to loosen it up.

8) Pour the balsamic reduction into the pan with the vegetables and mix until evenly coated.

9) Remove from heat and serve.

# Vegetable Soup

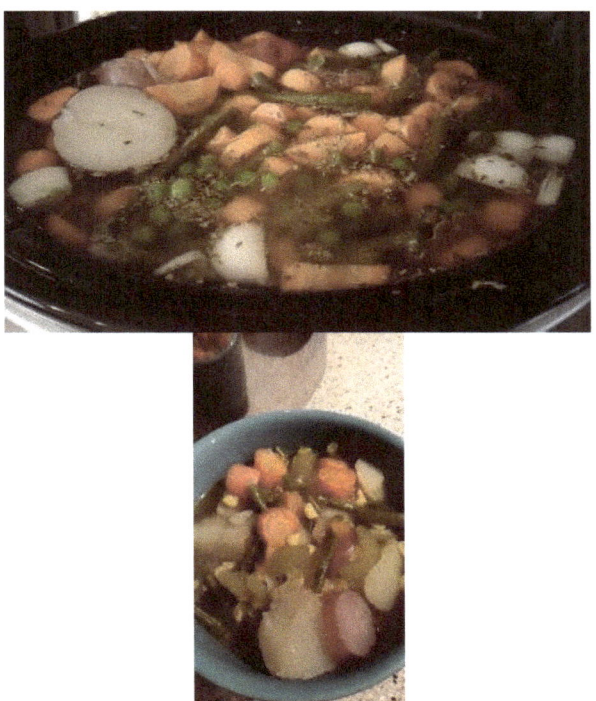

## Ingredients

- 3 carrots, sliced
- 4 stalks of celery, sliced
- 6 mushrooms, button or baby bellas,
- ½ of a large onion or one small onion, diced
- 2 cloves of garlic, minced
- 1 pound of fresh green beans
- 2 cups of cilantro
- 1 can of corn or 2 ears of corn, shaved
- 2 tablespoons Italian seasoning
- 2 bay leaves
- ½ cup sangria or chianti
- Water
- Salt and pepper to taste

## Instructions

1) Heat large pot over medium heat.
2) Add onion, carrot, and celery.
3) Stir constantly and heat over medium for about 3 minutes.
4) Pour wine into mixture and simmer until wine starts to evaporate.
5) Add the rest of the ingredients and water until it is just above the ingredients.
6) Bring to a boil.
7) Reduce heat and simmer, add more water if necessary.
8) Cook until the green beans are tender, and then serve.

Dressings, Sauces, & Toppings

# Avocado Dip

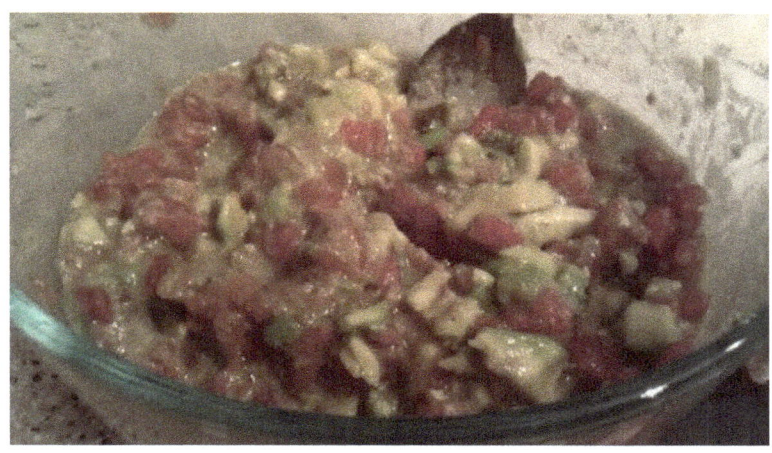

Serves 4
Prep time: 5 minutes

Ingredients
- 1 can Ro-tel or any type of spicy canned tomatoes
- 1 avocado
- ½ lime
- Salt & pepper to taste

Instructions
1) Pit one avocado and slice into small pieces and put in small mixing bowl.
2) With a fork, smash the avocado into small pieces.
3) Add Ro-tel.
4) Squeeze in half a lime.
5) Add salt & pepper to taste.
6) Serve immediately.

# Creamy Italian Dressing

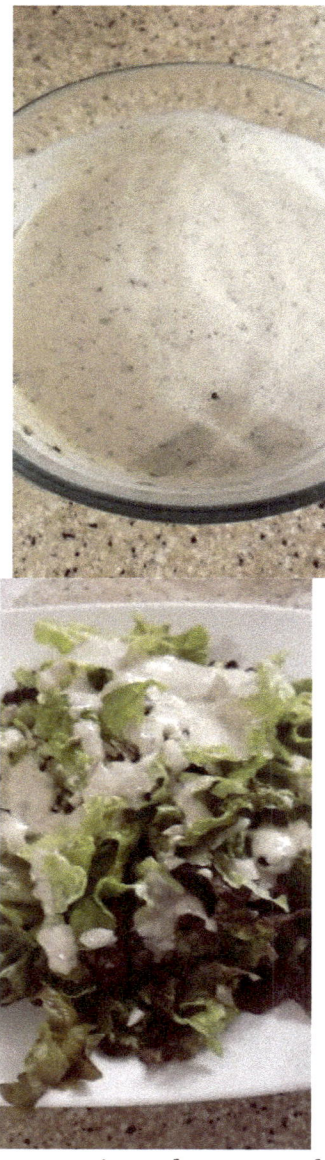

This recipe makes approximately 3 cups of dressing.

Ingredients

- 2 cups cashews
- Juice of 1 lime
- Salt to taste
- White pepper to taste
- Approximately 1 cup of water – add more by tablespoon until you reach desired consistency
- 1/4 teaspoon each dried ingredients ground together:
- Basil
- Oregano
- Rosemary
- Lemon pepper
- Garlic powder

Instructions
1) In a high-speed blender, add cashews, lime, salt, pepper and half of the water.
2) Blend, adding more water until desired consistency.
3) Pour mixture into a storage container and stir in the spices. Adjust spices to taste.
4) Refrigerate leftover dressing.

# Seasoned Nuts

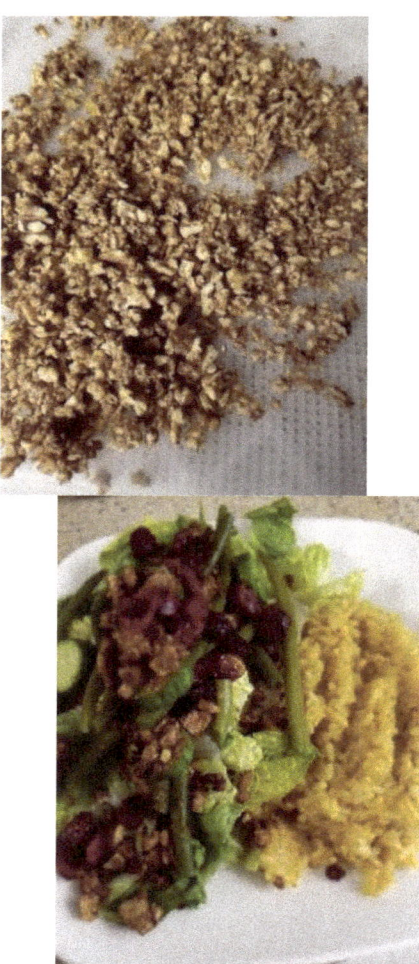

These nuts are a perfect topping for salads and other dishes.

Ingredients
- 2 cups chopped walnuts
- 1/4 cup cinnamon
- 2 tablespoons of maple syrup

Instructions
1) Mix ingredients
2) Dehydrate at 135 degrees for 8 hours in dehydrator
3) In the oven, roast on the lowest temperature and check after 30 minutes and roast until dry, checking every few minutes. These will burn quickly so check frequently.

# Drunken Mushrooms

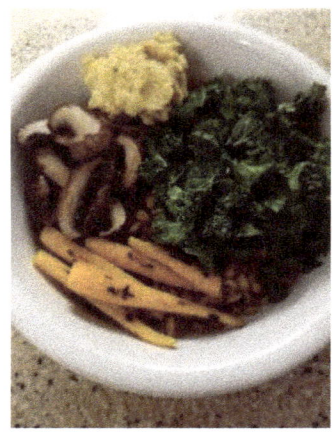 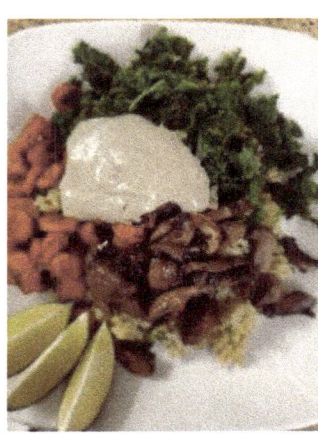

Ingredients
- Approximately 2 cups of mushrooms, washed and sliced
- ¼ cup red wine or vegetable stock
- Salt & pepper to taste

Instructions
1) Add mushrooms to a small pan with salt and pepper on medium heat. Stir occasionally.
2) When the mushrooms start to release their juices, add about ¼ cup of red wine and reduce to simmer, stirring occasionally, until mushrooms reach the desired texture.
3) Remove from heat and set aside in a small bowl.

NOTE! You can use vegetable stock instead of wine. The flavor won't be as savory, but it can be used as a substitute.

# Roasted Portobello Mushrooms

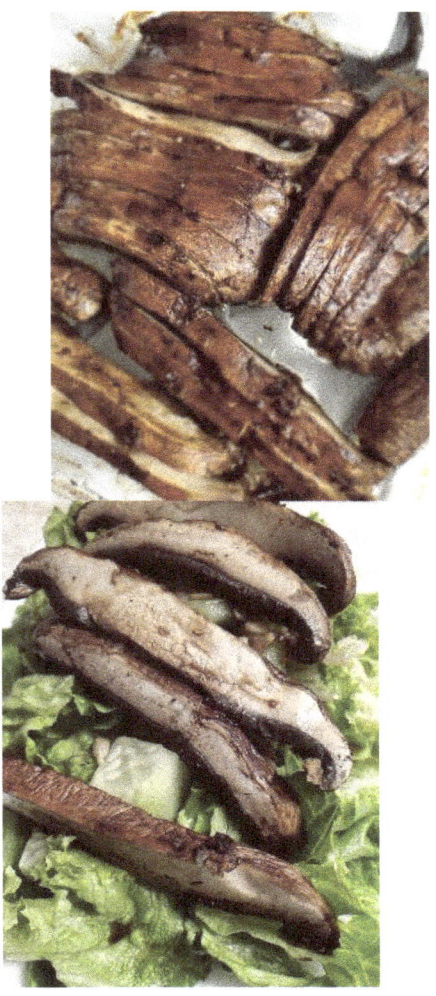

Ingredients
- 2 portobello mushrooms, sliced
- Balsamic vinegar
- Tamari
- Minced garlic
- Grated ginger
- Salt and pepper

Instructions
1) Preheat oven to 400
2) Mix all ingredients in a small bowl
3) Brush over sliced mushrooms
4) Bake 20 minutes
5) Serve over your favorite salad

# Sour Cream

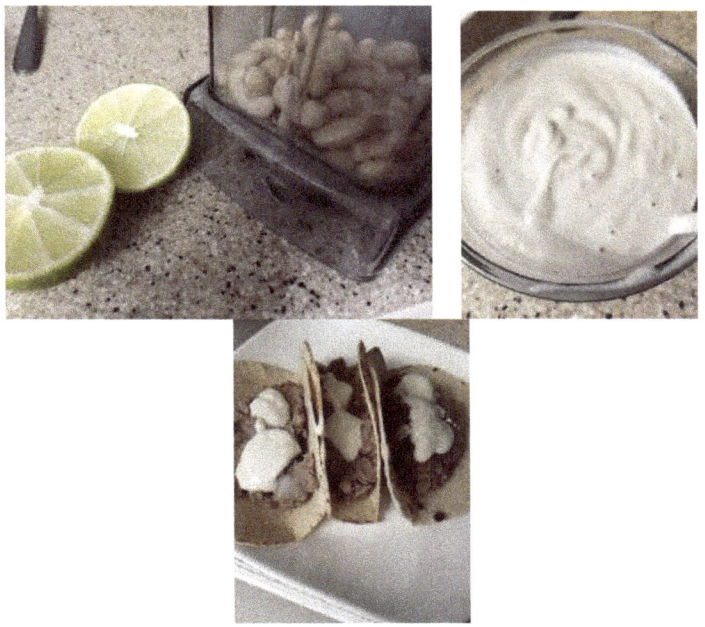

Ingredients
- 1 ½ cups cashews
- Juice of 2 limes
- Salt and pepper to taste
- Approximately 2 cups of water – add more until you reach desired consistency

Instructions
1) In a high-speed blender, add cashews, lime, salt, pepper, and half of the water.
2) Blend, adding more water until desired consistency.
3) Pour mixture into a storage container and refrigerate up to 4 days.

# VEGETABLE STOCK

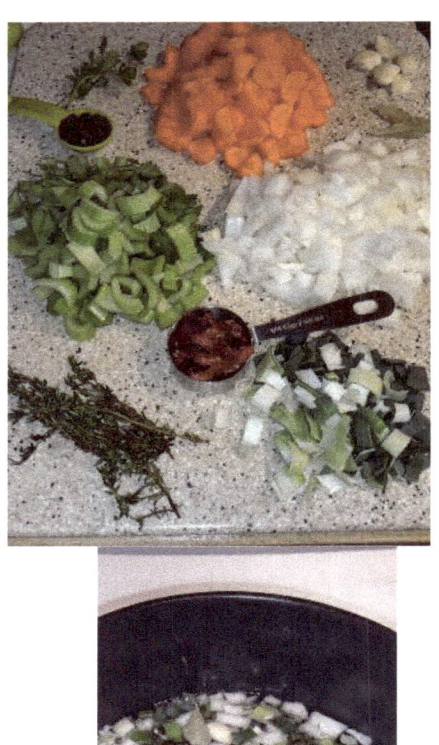

Ingredients

You can use quartered ingredients or sliced as in the picture.

- 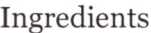 2 carrots

- 4 celery ribs
- 1 small onion
- 5 cloves garlic
- 3 leek leaves, washed
- 2 bay leaves
- Fresh rosemary, approximately 1/8 cup
- Fresh parsley, approximately 1/8 cup
- Fresh sage, approximately 1/8 cup
- Fresh thyme, approximately 1/8 cup
- 1 tablespoon whole peppercorns
- ¼ cup sundried tomatoes
- Salt to taste
- Approximately 20 cups of water

Add these after cooking stock.

- ¼ cup nutritional yeast
- 1 teaspoon ground turmeric
- 1 teaspoon smoked paprika

Instructions
1) Mix all ingredients for boiling in a large pot.
2) Bring to boil and reduce heat to simmer. Cover.
3) Simmer for approximately two hours or until it reaches desired flavor.
4) Using a strainer, strain the stock into a large bowl and toss out the vegetables. I put mine outside for the wildlife or add to a compost. Or, you can plan to make a vegetable soup right after the stock is prepared and add them to your soup at the end of cooking, just to heat them.
5) Stir in the yeast, turmeric, and smoked paprika.
6) Add to your favorite soups, pastas, or use to season mashed potatoes.
7) Store in a covered bowl in the refrigerator for 5 days.

# **Dessert**

# Blueberry Chia Seed Pudding

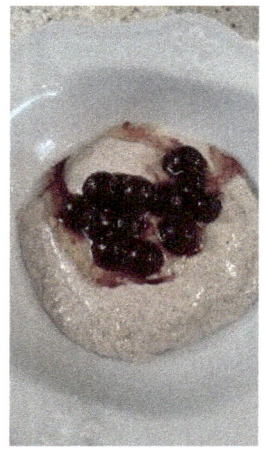 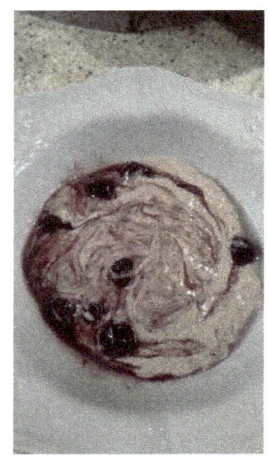

Ingredients

- 2 1/4 cups cashew milk
- 1/2 cup cashews
- 1/2 cup chia seeds
- 1 tsp vanilla
- 1 tablespoon cinnamon
- Dash of ground nutmeg
- 1/2 tsp pumpkin pie spice
- Blueberries for topping

Instructions

1) Put everything except for the blueberries in a high-speed blender until smooth.
2) Serve with blueberries or any other desired topping.
3) This pudding can be eaten for dessert or breakfast.

# Pumpkin Cashew Pudding

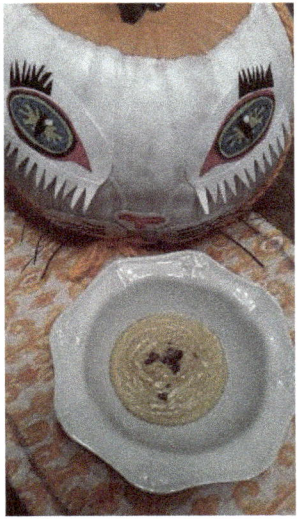
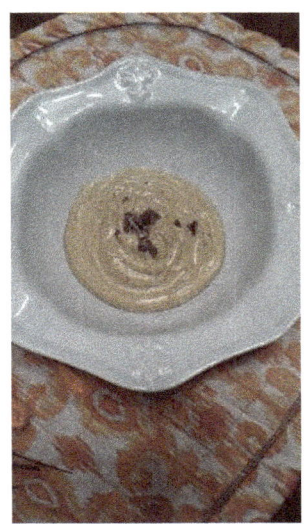

Ingredients

- 2 1/2 cups almond milk
- 1 cup cashews
- 1 tablespoon chia seeds
- 1 teaspoon vanilla
- 2 tablespoons arrowroot
- 1/2 of a 15 ounce can pumpkin puree (or sweet potato)
- 1/4 cup cacao nibs
- 6 medjool dates
- 1/2 teaspoon ground nutmeg
- 1 tablespoon cinnamon

Instructions

1) Add all ingredients in high-speed blender.
2) Blend for 1 to 2 minutes or until smooth. You may have to use the tamper because it's thick.
3) Pour into a bowl, chill, and serve with fresh grated nutmeg and cacao nibs, if desired.

# Quinoa Balls

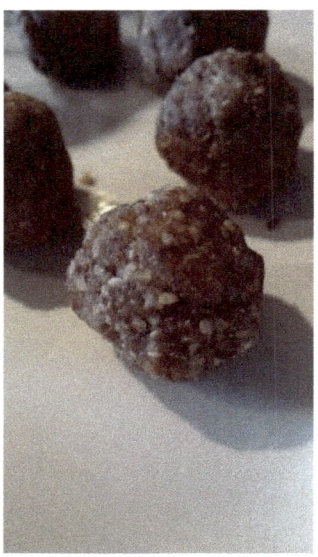

Ingredients

- 4 pitted medjool dates
- 1/2 cup figs
- 1 cup crushed walnuts
- 1/4 cup sesame seeds
- 1/2 tsp almond extract
- 1/2 tsp vanilla
- Pinch of sea salt
- Dash of all spice
- 1/4 cup quinoa flour

Instructions

1) Add everything to food processor for 2 minutes.
2) Form into approximately 10 balls and serve
3) Store in an airtight container on the counter for up to 3 days or in the freezer for up to 1 month.

# Healthy Vegan Strawberry Crumble

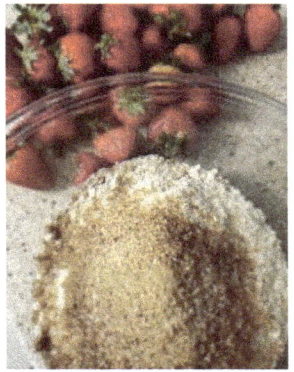
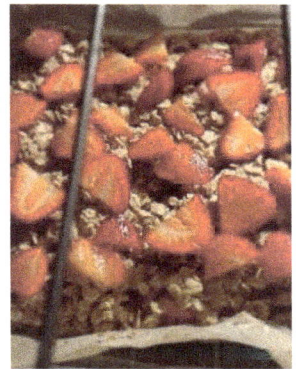
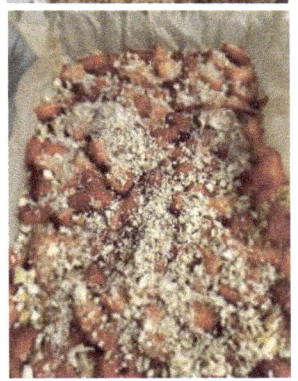
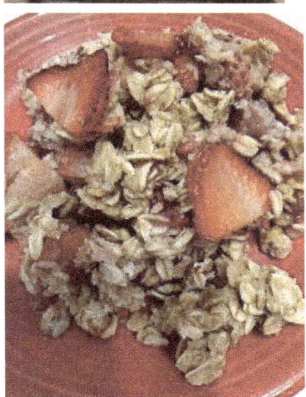

Ingredients

- 3 cups rolled oats
- 2 cups almond flour
- 1/2 cup raw sugar
- 1/2 teaspoon ground ginger
- 1/2 teaspoon fresh grated nutmeg
- Dash of salt

Instructions
1) Preheat oven to 375.

2) Mix these ingredients in a large bowl.
3) After mixing dry ingredients, add approximately 1 cup oat milk or just enough to make mixture crumbly.
4) Line a 9 x13 inch baking dish with parchment paper.
5) Wash and dice around 3 cups of strawberries. Reserve about 1 cup for top.
6) Put half of crumble mixture in pan and pat it down with your hands.
7) Top with diced strawberries.
8) Optional, chop about 1/2 cup of almonds into crumble. Sprinkle on top of strawberries.
9) Top strawberries with other half of crumble mixture.
10) Bake for 15 minutes.
11) While baking, slice remaining strawberries and cover mix with juice of one lemon and 1 tablespoon of raw sugar.
12) Remove from oven and add strawberries to the top.
13) Bake an additional 15 minutes.
14) Allow it to cool before serving.

# Strawberry Cacao Pudding and Strawberry Paste

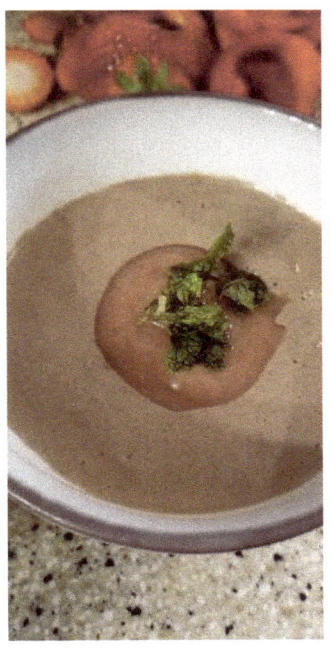 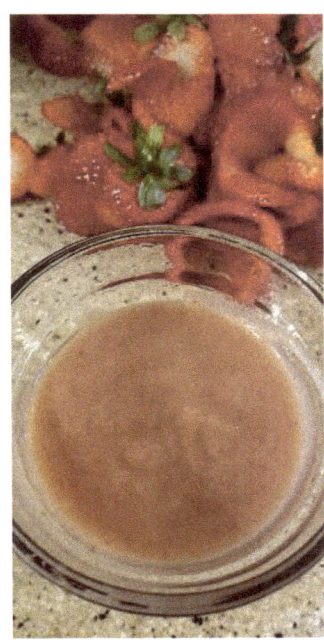

Pudding Ingredients
- 10 to 12 peeled strawberries
- 1 cup cashews
- 2 1/2 cups of your favorite non-dairy milk
- 2 tablespoons chia seeds
- 1 teaspoon vanilla
- 2 tablespoons cacao powder
- 6 to 8 medjool dates (add to your desired sweetness)

Instructions
1) For the pudding, add the following ingredients into a high-speed blender.

2) Blend, taste, and add more milk alternative if necessary, 1/4 cup at a time, until creamy and no longer chalky.
3) Refrigerate for one to two hours or until set, preferably overnight.
4) Enjoy with fresh mint leaves and strawberry paste.

For strawberry paste, add the following ingredients into a high-speed blender.

- 10 to 12 peeled strawberries
- 2 medjool dates
- 1 teaspoon vanilla

Blend until smooth.

Store in an airtight container in the refrigerator for up to 5 days.

Enjoy with pudding or use as a spread on toast or waffles.

# INDEX

Apple, 35
Arthritis, 19, 84, 110
Artichoke, 34
Asthma, 17, 87, 106
Autoimmune, 38
Avocado, 34, 315
B1, 46
B-12, 42, 44, 45, 46
B6, 46, 104
Barrette's esophagus, 17
B-carotene, 28
Beans, 14, 28, 32, 33, 34, 35, 37, 54, 74, 130, 163, 167, 181, 277, 278, 279, 283, 284, 285, 291, 295, 296, 307, 308, 311, 312, 313, 314
Beta-carotene, 37
Bioavailability, 129
Blackberries, 35
Blood pressure, 49, 55, 56, 57, 68, 72, 83, 87, 91, 96, 106, 115, 117
Blood sugar, 74, 75, 87, 89
Blueberries, 69, 70, 326
Bran, 32, 34, 36, 46
Butyrates, 38
Cacao, 70, 71, 72, 167, 331
Calcium, 37, 91, 118, 121, 126, 127, 128, 129, 130, 131
Cancer, 16, 18, 24, 25, 26, 27, 28, 31, 38, 42, 44, 45, 61, 62, 63, 64, 68, 78, 89, 91, 108, 112, 114, 131, 161, 162
Cardiovascular, 24, 28, 54, 78, 110

Casein, 121, 132
Cashews, 102, 167
Cereal, 28, 32, 33, 34, 43, 73, 95, 97
Chia seeds, 35, 167
Cholesterol, 37, 50
Cinnamon, 73, 75
Circulation, 70, 87, 129
Complex carbohydrates, 38, 39
Complex regional pain syndrome, 18
Coronary artery disease, 49, 56, 89
Cow, 14, 118, 129, 132
Cranberry, 33
Crohn's, 108, 135, 136, 137
CRPS, 18
Cruciferous vegetables, 76, 78
Dehydration, 115
Depression, 13, 16, 162
Diabetes, 15, 16, 24, 25, 30, 47, 49, 51, 61, 75, 96, 101, 111, 112, 142, 157, 161
Diabetes, 13
Dyslexia, 133
Energy, 45, 63, 111, 115
Erythromelalgia, 18, 94
Fat, 37, 121
Fennel, 80, 81
Figs, 35
Folate, 37
Garlic, 82, 317
Ginger, 84
Glucose, 55
Glycemic index, 47

Green Tea, 88
HDL, 51, 52, 53, 55, 57
Heart, 13, 16, 17, 24, 25,
26, 27, 31, 49, 50, 51,
52, 53, 54, 55, 56, 58,
59, 60, 61, 67, 71, 72,
83, 87, 96, 112, 127,
131, 134, 157, 161, 162
Heart disease, 13, 16, 17,
24, 25, 26, 27, 31, 49,
50, 54, 58, 59, 60, 61,
67, 71, 83, 87, 96, 112,
131, 161, 162
High blood cholesterol,
49
Hypertension, 24, 67
Hypoglycemia, 17, 52
Inflammation, 38, 50, 56,
71, 78, 84, 87, 104, 110
Iron, 37
Irritable Bowel
Syndrome, 39
Ischemic heart disease,
67
Kidney, 118, 285, 291
Lacto-ovo vegetarians, 63
Lactose intolerant, 118
LDL, 51, 52, 53, 55, 56,
57, 72
Leafy greens, 90, 91
Lentils, 33, 182
Lipoproteins, 53
Liver, 50, 51, 53, 108
Low-fat, 16, 55, 109, 111,
142
Lupus, 17, 18
Magnesium, 37, 121
Mental health, 111, 162
Multiple sclerosis, 70,
109, 162
Multivitamin, 27

Nonheme iron, 118
Nutrition, 17, 19, 21, 25,
26, 31, 43, 46, 50, 61,
64, 65, 82, 91, 95, 119,
128, 130, 133, 134, 161
Nutritionist, 66
Obesity, 13, 24, 49, 51
Oil
oil, 121, 142
Omega-3 fatty acids, 53,
54
Osteoarthritis, 110
Osteoporosis, 126, 127,
128
Pancreatic, 78
Pear, 34
Peas, 28, 33, 34, 35, 37,
167, 271, 272, 281, 282,
304, 305
Peppermint, 93
Postural orthostatic
tachycardia syndrome,
POTS, 18
Protein, 9, 22, 23, 28, 32,
38, 42, 47, 52, 53, 54,
56, 61, 62, 63, 66, 71,
91, 96, 102, 104, 109,
110, 118, 129, 131, 155,
158, 161, 262
Proteins, 28, 96, 109
Pumpkin, 34, 36, 275,
301, 327
Quinoa, 37, 95, 96, 167,
271, 328
Raspberries, 35
Raynaud's, 18
Reflexive sympathetic
dystrophy, RSD, 18, 75
sympathetic, 18, 115
Rheumatoid arthritis, 17
Sage, 98, 99

Seeds, 34, 77, 80, 81, 95, 96, 100, 101, 103, 130, 135, 155, 264, 275, 282, 301, 326, 327, 328, 331
Short chain fatty acid, 38
Sjogren's, 17
Soybeans, 34, 35
Standard American Diet, 21, 31
Stroke, 39, 53, 54, 68, 72

Supplement, 26, 28, 30, 42, 44, 45, 127, 128
Sweet potato, 35
Sweet potatoes, 103
Thyme, 105, 106
Turmeric, 107, 108, 268
Vegetarians, 22, 23, 24, 54, 57, 64, 125, 154
Vitamin, 26, 27, 37
Vitamin C, 27, 42, 56
Vitamin E, 26, 27, 28, 96

# SOURCES

[1] Toumpanakis, Turnbull, & Alba-Barba, Effectiveness of plant-based diets in promoting well-being in the management of type 2 diabetes: a systematic review (bmj.com): Le & Sabate, Beyond meatless, the health effects of vegan diets: findings from the Adventist cohorts - PubMed (nih.gov)

[2] Hever, Plant-Based Diets: A Physician's Guide - PubMed (nih.gov)

[3] (See 1)

[4] (See 1)

[5] (See 4)

[6] (See 1)

[7] Touzeau et al., Diet of Ancient Egyptians inferred from stable isotope systematics

[8] (See 9)

[9] (See 9)

[10] Clarys et al., Comparison of nutritional quality of the vegan, vegetarian, semi-vegetarian, pesco-vegetarian and omnivorous diet - PubMed (nih.gov)

[11] (See 12)

[12] National Agricultural Library, 2011

[13] United States Department of Agriculture, n.d.

[14] Le & Sabate, Beyond meatless, the health effects of vegan diets: findings from the Adventist cohorts - PubMed (nih.gov)

[15] Reinhart, 2019

[16] (See 16)

[17] National Center for Health Statistics [NCHS], 2017; Tuso, Stoll, & Li, 2015; Physician's Committee for Responsible Medicine, 2019; Center for Disease Control and Prevention, 2015

[18] (See 16)

[19] Satija et al., Plant-Based Dietary Patterns and Incidence of Type 2 Diabetes in US Men and Women: Results from Three Prospective Cohort Studies (plos.org)

[20] Rahman, Implementation of a Plant-Based, Nutrition Program in a Large Integrated Health Care System: Results of a Pilot Program (nih.gov)

[21] Wakim, Ritchey, Hockenberry, & Casper, Geographic Variations in Incremental Costs of Heart Disease Among Medicare Beneficiaries, by Type of Service, 2012 - PubMed (nih.gov)

[22] O'Neil et al., Relationship between diet and mental health in children and adolescents: a systematic review - PubMed (nih.gov)

[23] Mobbs et. al, The ecology of human fear: survival optimization and the nervous system (nih.gov)

[24] Blumenschine, 1987, (PDF) Hunting and Scavenging by Early Humans: The State of the Debate | StAte Debate - Academia.edu

[25] Kamangar & Emadi, Vitamin and mineral supplements: do we really need them? - PubMed (nih.gov)

[26] (See 27)

[27] The alpha-tocopherol, beta-carotene lung cancer prevention study: Design, methods, participant characteristics, and compliance, Annals of Epidemiology, Volume 4, Issue 1, 1994, Pages 1-10, ISSN 1047-2797, https://doi.org/10.1016/1047-2797(94)90036-1.

[28] Kamangar, F., & Emadi, A. (2012). Vitamin and mineral supplements: do we really need them?. *International journal of preventive medicine*, *3*(3), 221–226.

[29] Sesso, H. D., Buring, J. E., Christen, W. G., Kurth, T., Belanger, C., MacFadyen, J., Bubes, V., Manson, J. E., Glynn, R. J., & Gaziano, J. M. (2008). Vitamins E and C in the prevention of cardiovascular disease in men: the Physicians' Health Study II randomized controlled trial. *JAMA*, *300*(18), 2123–2133. https://doi.org/10.1001/jama.2008.600

[30] Lee, I. M., Cook, N. R., Gaziano, J. M., Gordon, D., Ridker, P. M., Manson, J. E., Hennekens, C. H., & Buring, J. E. (2005). Vitamin E in the primary prevention of cardiovascular disease and cancer: the Women's Health Study: a randomized controlled trial. *JAMA*, *294*(1), 56–65. https://doi.org/10.1001/jama.294.1.56

[31] Delimaris, Adverse Effects Associated with Protein Intake above the Recommended Dietary Allowance for Adults - PubMed (nih.gov)

[32] Ward, 1937; Bureau of Human Nutrition and Home Economics, 1944, Records of the Bureau of Human Nutrition and Home Economics | National Archives

[33] (See 34)

[34] Hu, E. A., Pan, A., Malik, V., & Sun, Q. (2012). White rice consumption and risk of type 2 diabetes: meta-analysis and systematic review. The BMJ, 344, e1454. http://doi.org/10.1136/bmj.e1454

[35] Office of Disease Prevention and Health Promotion. (2015). *Current Eating Patterns in the United States*. Retrieved on January 3, 2019 from

https://health.gov/dietaryguidelines/2015/guidelines/chapter-2/current-eating-patterns-in-the-united-states/

[36] (See 38)

[37] Centers for Disease Control and Prevention. (2017, March). *Leading causes of death.* Retrieved December 29, 2018 from https://www.cdc.gov/nchs/fastats/leading-causes-of-death.htm

[38] Office of Disease Prevention and Health Promotion. (2015). *Current Eating Patterns in the United States.* Retrieved on January 3, 2019 from https://health.gov/dietaryguidelines/2015/guidelines/chapter-2/current-eating-patterns-in-the-united-states/

[39] The National Academies of Sciences Engineering Medicine. (2002). *Dietary Reference Intakes for Energy, Carbohydrate, Fiber, Fat, Fatty Acids, Cholesterol, Protein, and Amino Acids.* Retrieved on January 4, 2019 from http://www.nationalacademies.org/hmd/Reports/2002/Dietary-Reference-Intakes-for-Energy-Carbohydrate-Fiber-Fat-Fatty-Acids-Cholesterol-Protein-and-Amino-Acids.aspx

[40] Office of Disease Prevention and Health Promotion. (2014). *Food Sources of Dietary Fiber.* Retrieved January 3, 2019 from https://health.gov/dietaryguidelines/2015/guidelines/appendix-13/

[41] Chiba, M., Tsuda, S., Komatsu, M., Tozawa, H., & Takayama, Y. (2016). Onset of Ulcerative Colitis during a Low-Carbohydrate Weight-Loss Diet and Treatment with a Plant-Based Diet: A Case Report. *The Permanente journal, 20*(1), 80-4.

[42] Canani, R. B., Costanzo, M. D., Leone, L., Pedata, M., Meli, R., & Calignano, A. (2011). Potential beneficial effects of butyrate in intestinal and extraintestinal diseases. *World journal of gastroenterology, 17*(12), 1519-28.

[43] Canani, R. B., Costanzo, M. D., Leone, L., Pedata, M., Meli, R., & Calignano, A. (2011). Potential beneficial effects of butyrate in intestinal and extraintestinal diseases. *World journal of gastroenterology, 17*(12), 1519-28.

[44] Chiba, M., Tsuda, S., Komatsu, M., Tozawa, H., & Takayama, Y. (2016). Onset of Ulcerative Colitis during a Low-Carbohydrate Weight-Loss Diet and Treatment with a Plant-Based Diet: A Case Report. *The Permanente journal, 20*(1), 80-4.

[45] Lea, Crawford, & Worsley, Consumers' readiness to eat a plant-based diet - PubMed (nih.gov)

[46] Craig, Health effects of vegan diets - PubMed (nih.gov)

[47] Campbell, T. Colin Campbell Center for Nutrition Studies

[48] Richter et al., Plant protein and animal proteins: do they differentially affect cardiovascular disease risk? - PubMed (nih.gov)

[49] (See 49)

[50] Office of Dietary Supplements, Office of Dietary Supplements (ODS) (nih.gov)

[51] Office of Dietary Supplements

[52] Campbell, T. Colin Campbell Center for Nutrition Studies

[53] (See 55).

[54] (Brasky, White, & Chen, 2017)

[55] https://www.gardenoflife.com/content/product/mykind-organics-vegan-b-12-organic-spray/

[56] Slavin et al., Why whole grains are protective: biological mechanisms (cambridge.org)

[57] Centers for Disease Control and Prevention [CDC], 2019

[58] United States Census Bureau, 2020; CDC, 2019

[59] Kerley, 2018

[60] Width, M. & Reinhard, T. (2021). *The essential pocket guide for clinical nutrition.* Burlington, MA: Jones & Bartlett Learning. p. 392

[61] https://ods.od.nih.gov/factsheets/Omega3FattyAcids-HealthProfessional/

[62] Kerley, C. P. (2018). A Review of Plant-based Diets to Prevent and Treat Heart Failure. *Cardiac Failure Review*, 4(1), 54–61. http://doi.org/10.15420/cfr.2018:1:1

[63] (See 66)

[64] (See 66)

[65] (See 66)

[66] Yokoyama Y, Nishimura K, Barnard ND, et al. Vegetarian Diets and Blood PressureA Meta-analysis. *JAMA Intern Med.* 2014;174(4):577–587. doi:10.1001/jamainternmed.2013.14547

[67] (See 69)

[68] Pettersen et al., Vegetarian diets and blood pressure among white subjects: results from the Adventist Health Study-2 (AHS-2) - PubMed (nih.gov)

[69] Weggemans, Zock, & Katan, Dietary cholesterol from eggs increases the ratio of total cholesterol to high-density lipoprotein cholesterol in humans: A meta-analysis

[70] American Heart Association, 2019
[71] Oklahoma Heart Hospital, 2019
[72] Campbell & Campbell, The China Study
[73] Campbell & Campbell, The China Study
[74] Campbell & Campbell, The China Study
[75] (See 75)
[76] (See 75)
[77] (See 75)
[78] Orlich MJ, Singh PN, Sabaté J, et al. Vegetarian Dietary Patterns and the Risk of Colorectal Cancers. *JAMA Intern Med.* 2015;175(5):767–776. doi:10.1001/jamainternmed.2015.59

[79] American Cancer Society, 2016
[80] Slavin et al., Why whole grains are protective: biological mechanisms (cambridge.org)
[81] Adams, K. M., Kohlmeier, M., & Zeisel, S. H. (2010). Nutrition education in U.S. medical schools: latest update of a national survey. *Academic medicine : journal of the Association of American Medical Colleges, 85*(9), 1537-42.
[82] (See 84)
[83] (See 22)
[84] Hughes, G. J., Kress, K. S., Armbrecht, E. S., Mukherjea, R., & Mattfeldt-Beman, M. (2014). Initial investigation of dietitian perception of plant-based protein quality. *Food Science & Nutrition, 2*(4), 371–379. http://doi.org/10.1002/fsn3.112

[85] Wakim et al., Geographic Variations in Incremental Costs of Heart Disease Among Medicare Beneficiaries, by Type of Service, 2012 (cdc.gov)
[86] (See 88)
[87] Chronic Conditions Data Warehouse, 2020
[88] National Center for Chronic Disease Prevention and Health Promotion 2019
[89] (See 22)
[90] Myths About Diet and Your Thyroid | Northwestern Medicine

[91] Proceedings of the National Academy of Sciences of the United States of America (2017, November). *Early Neolithic Wine of Georgia in the South Caucasus.* Retrieved August 7, 2019 from https://www.pnas.org/content/114/48/E10309

[92] Dark Green Leafy Vegetables : USDA ARS

[93] A Sweet Potato History | Inside Adams: Science, Technology & Business (loc.gov)

[94] Swank, Treatment of multiple sclerosis with low-fat diet - PubMed (nih.gov)

[95] Swank & Dugan, Effect of low saturated fat diet in early and late cases of multiple sclerosis - ScienceDirect

[96] Yadav et al., Low-fat, plant-based diet in multiple sclerosis: A randomized controlled trial - PubMed (nih.gov)

[97] Clinton et al., Whole-foods, plant-based diet alleviates the symptoms of osteoarthritis - PubMed (nih.gov)

[98] Satija et al., Plant-Based Dietary Patterns and Incidence of Type 2 Diabetes in US Men and Women: Results from Three Prospective Cohort Studies (plos.org)

[99] O'Neil et al., Relationship between diet and mental health in children and adolescents: a systematic review - PubMed (nih.gov)

[100] Mayo Clinic, 2019

[101] Vij, V. A., & Joshi, A. S. (2013). Effect of 'water induced thermogenesis' on body weight, body mass index and body composition of overweight subjects. *Journal of clinical and diagnostic research : JCDR*, 7(9), 1894–1896. https://doi.org/10.7860/JCDR/2013/5862.3344

[102] Vij, V. A., & Joshi, A. S. (2013). Effect of 'water induced thermogenesis' on body weight, body mass index and body composition of overweight subjects. *Journal of clinical and diagnostic research : JCDR*, 7(9), 1894–1896. https://doi.org/10.7860/JCDR/2013/5862.3344

[103] Armstrong, L. & Johnson, E. (2018). Water intake, water balance, and the elusive daily water requirement. *Nutrients.* Doi: 10.3390/nu10121928

[104] https://www.pcrm.org/good-nutrition/nutrition-information/health-concerns-about-dairy/calcium-and-strong-bones

[105] Milk Allergy - Dr. Manik G. Hiranandani (drmanik.net)

[106] How Bacteria In Cows' Milk May Cause Crohn's Disease -- ScienceDaily

[107] Why does the diet eliminate oil entirely? | Dr. Esselstyn's Prevent & Reverse Heart Disease Program (dresselstyn.com)

[108] World Population is Three Times the Sustainable Level. World Population Balance. (2013). Retrieved on November 3, 2013 from http://www.worldpopulationbalance.org/3_times_sustainable.

[109] University of Florida. (2006). Living Green. Retrieved November 3, 2013 from http://livinggreen.ifas.ufl.edu/.

[110] Sustainable Earth,
Green Diets: Change Your Diet and Help the Earth. (2013). Retrieved on November 3, 2013 from http://www.isustainableearth.com/sustainable-living/green-diets-help-the-earth.

[111] Starr, C., Evers, C.A., Starr, L. (2008). *Biology: Concepts and Applications*. Belmont, CA: Thompson Books.

[112] Road to Rio +20. (2011). Retrieved November 3, 2013 from United Nations at http://www.uncsd2012.org/

[113] Brown, P. (2013). Sustainable Living Challenges the Swiss. Retrieved November 3, 2013 from Truth Dig at http://www.truthdig.com/report/item/sustainable_living_challenges_the_swiss_20130528.

[114] Cho, R. (2013). Just How Effective is Green Infrastructure? Retrieved November 3, 2013 from Columbia at http://blogs.ei.columbia.edu/2013/10/31/just-how-effective-is-green-infrastructure/.

# About the Author

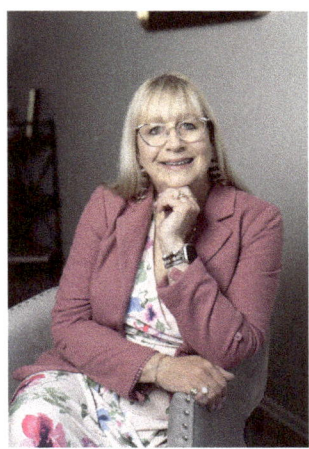

Jody Ortiz has written over 100 books since she began her career as a ghost writer in 2004. She is certified in plant-based nutrition through Cornell's online program, has trained as a professional plant-based chef, and holds a Bachelor's Degree in Liberal Arts from The University of Oklahoma.

In 2020, she stepped into the coaching world and graduated as a miracle-minded vegan coach, trained by spiritual leader and former presidential candidate, Marianne Williamson.

By day, she works as a vegan chef and miracle-minded vegan coach. By night, she pens her own series of books in the true crime, non-fiction, children, and adult fiction genres.

She currently lives in Oklahoma with her husband and daughter as well as 19 winged, scaled, and four-legged family members. Her hobbies include spending time with her family members, cooking, knitting, sewing, playing viola, writing (she loves what she does), and giving a voice to the cause that is close to her heart, wrongful convictions.

You can find out more about her by visiting www.jodyortiz.com.